IN FITNESS AND IN HEALTH

A practical guide
to healthy diet
and nutrition,
exercise, injury
prevention
and avoiding
disease

Dr. Philip Maffetone

REVISED AND EXPANDED FIFTH EDITION

In Fitness and In Health

*A Practical Guide to Healthy Diet and Nutrition,
Exercise, Injury Prevention and Avoiding Disease*

Fifth Revised Edition

© 2009 Dr. Philip Maffetone
All rights reserved

Editor: Hal Walter
Cover Design: Cheri Zanotelli
Text Design and Typography: Out There

Printed in the United States
Library of Congress Control Number: 2001012345
ISBN: 1-4392-3282-2

The information contained in this book is from the author's experiences and is not intended to replace medical advice. It is not the intent of the author to diagnose or prescribe.

Before beginning any program you should consult with your physician, and address any questions to your physician.

Case studies in this book are those of real people whose names have been changed to protect confidentiality.

Table of Contents

"Now I see the secret of the making of the best persons. It is to grow in the open air, and to eat and sleep with the earth."

— Walt Whitman, *Leaves of Grass*

Introduction

With this new edition of "In Fitness and In Health," it's more obvious than ever that we have entered a new era in health care. The responsibility for personal health has shifted from a broken health-care system back to each of us. It's a time when we demand higher quality of life now and for the future. In this age of true prevention, we seek to avoid the illnesses we almost accept as part of the aging process. We want to postpone — effectively preventing — cancer, heart disease and Alzheimer's rather than settle for early detection. We would rather be full of life in our "golden years" than spend a decade or more at the end of life in dysfunction. The tools to do this are contained in this newly rewritten and expanded fifth edition.

I continue sharing my experiences on improving health as a balance of art and science. This stems from my clinical practice in complementary medicine, which began in 1977, and — previous to that — being a patient. The art facet entails a unique understanding of both fitness and health. I compiled the actual science through my early education, then extensive clinical research. In this book I combine this art with this science in hopes of helping you to fully understand and simplify many of the complex mechanisms of fitness and health.

I have worked with patients from all walks of life, from the most healthy to the most frail, from professional athletes to couch potatoes. Many had unique imbalances that not only caused dysfunction, but detracted from their quality of life, reducing what I call "human performance." Many of these problems were the result of dietary and nutritional imbalances, and others stemmed from deficiencies in the aerobic system or the stress-coping mechanisms. It was clear that addressing these problems immediately and individually was the key not only to improving health in the short term, but also avoiding serious disease in the long run.

This reorganized and extensively updated edition addresses steps you can take to improve your health and fitness for a better quality of life now, and a longer life and higher human performance in your later years. It opens by defining key issues, terms and philosophies important in understanding how to achieve a balance of health and fitness, and optimal human performance. Since your health is so dependent upon the food you eat, this book extensively discusses food and nutrition, with some of the material challenging many long-held popular beliefs. Exercise is basic not only to fitness but also to health, and thus several chapters of this book discuss developing or modifying physical activity that is most appropriate for your needs. Lastly, the final chapters on self-health management tie together all the wisdom in the book. Included is the newest information that is scientifically based and clinically relevant, presented in a user-friendly format, with specific actions you can take to understand and prevent the most dangerous diseases facing modern humankind. By correcting and diverting seemingly subtle problems, you can prevent disease, modify the aging process, and drastically improve the quality of your life. We have more control over our health — through food, nutrition, stress control, exercise and other factors — than ever imagined. The remedies for the greatest of ailments have been with us all along. By redirecting and rethinking your responsibility in health care, you can immediately begin reaping the benefits.

With all the changes through these five editions of "In Fitness and In Health," the basic principles are the same as when the very first version of this book was created in the early 1980s. Then, talking about "good fats" and "bad carbohydrates" was blasphemy, and "easy exercise" was difficult to explain in an era of "no pain, no gain."

Most of these old tenants are being put aside by science, yet many continue to thrive in the public eye because tradition is so powerful. But along the way, many authors and companies started promoting similar ideas, programs and products (and some were essentially copies of what I presented). I am always happy to see the sharing of ideas since the ultimate goal is to help people achieve optimal health and fitness.

While many so-called health programs and diets come and go there is no one approach for everyone, except one that teaches how to individualize health and fitness to meet each of our unique needs. This book will help you do just that — determine which lifestyle factors best match your particular needs. By the end of the book you will know not only how to live most healthfully, and full of enjoyment, but also how to die most successfully.

You'll want to read this book from beginning to end, then continuously refer to it. Each time you read from it you'll understand more about your particular needs. In doing so, you'll want to share the information with friends and family, perhaps influencing others in their quest for better health and fitness.

Good health and fitness forever!

— *Dr. Phil Maffetone*

1

Defining Fitness and Health

It was the summer of 1976, and I wanted to watch the Olympic sprinters in Montreal. I was in a hospital bed with an undiagnosed illness that caused me to drop 60 pounds in less than a year. Now, weighing only 97 pounds, I was barely able to reach the switch for the TV and too weak to turn it on. The nurse came in to help me. While watching the Olympic games, I remembered the days when I was a national-class sprinter. And I wondered how my health could so rapidly deteriorate.

The road to full recovery from that illness was long, and required that I learn more about how my body works. In a sense I'm still on that road, continually and now intuitively assessing my food, nutrition, physical activity and lifestyle in order to stay healthy. By tuning in more closely to my body's needs after my illness I began to see the immediate benefits of improved health and also began to feel well for the first time in several years. During this period I began going for a walk every day. In April 1980, I found myself admiring the finishers of the Boston Marathon, thinking that these runners must be really healthy in order to run more than 26 miles. As I watched the marathoners finish I developed a desire to test my own health. I had been walking regularly for more than two years. The New York City Marathon was six months away and that seemed like plenty of time to train for it. After all, I mused, I ran in high school and in college.

It was a cool, overcast morning as I began my journey to the New York City Marathon. The race started with a cannon blast so loud it shook the Verrazano Bridge. The crowd of 18,000 runners began to move and I was among them, ready to prove to myself that I really was healthy. All went well through the first 10 miles. The excitement swept me along at a slightly quicker pace than planned, yet I felt great. As expected, by 15 miles I felt tired but was able to continue.

Within the next couple of miles, however, I began to shiver. Despite drinking plenty of water, I felt dehydrated. And I was craving cotton candy. At 18 miles, I stopped to check my feet. They were numb, and I wanted to be sure they were still there. "My hamstrings are cramping," I said out loud. Suddenly I realized I wasn't thinking rationally and all I could remember was my goal to finish the race and prove my health.

Alarmed by how bad I looked, two paramedics tried to take me off the course. But I wouldn't stop. Somehow, I fought my way onward. I have very little memory of those last few miles, but I'll always remember the finale. A minor collision with a TV camera in Central Park made me realize I was close to the end of the race. As the pain became more intense, the crowds got louder, and I finally had a clear view — the finish line.

A medal was hung around my neck, and I cried. I thought the lesson was over, but would soon be struck by a more meaningful one. The next moment I discovered myself in the first-aid tent. It looked like a war zone. There were casualties all around me. Doctors and nurses were running around. People on cots groaned in pain. Ambulances came and went.

Looking around I had to wonder: "Are these people really healthy?" I realized then that running the marathon had not proven my health at all. I was fit enough to run 26.2 miles. But clearly fitness was something quite different from health. The next morning, sore but happy, I pondered my new goal to improve my health. Achieving this would not be so simple as running a marathon. Optimal health would be something that I would continually strive to attain for the rest of my life.

The real lesson from my marathon experience was not one of proving health, but rather that I became fit enough to run a marathon. Clearly this had nothing to do with my health. Fitness and health, though many think the terms are interchangeable, are actually two different, but mutually dependent states.

Later, in treating patients who were very athletic, I would see individuals who were very fit but at the same time unhealthy; injuries, illness and other unhealthy conditions often accompanied their quests to be faster or go farther. Clearly, some athletes would be healthier had they stayed couch potatoes! On the other hand, I saw many sedentary people who attempted to get healthy without an adequate level of fitness — also a condition that was not ideal. The main reason for the dysfunction in both types of patient is an imbalance between fitness and health. Let us define these two important terms as follows:

Fitness: The ability to perform physical activity. You define the limits of your fitness; you can walk a mile a day or train for the Ironman Triathlon.

Health: The optimal balance of all systems of the body — the nervous, muscular, skeletal, circulatory, digestive, lymphatic, hormonal and all other systems.

Improving fitness is associated with physical activity. Only a couple of generations ago, most people were naturally active, working hard physically to accomplish their daily chores. Today, we have escalators, microwaves and remote controls. Some people drive around a parking lot for 10 minutes to get a parking space closer to the door. Others wait minutes for an elevator just to go to the first floor. We can fulfill most of our needs literally at the push of a button. This radical change from a vigorous to an inactive lifestyle has taken place, genetically speaking, in a very short time frame. The human body can't adapt to such a major change without dire consequences. Our relative inactivity has resulted in an overweight and obese society and an entire host of other functional disorders from blood-sugar problems and overfat bodies, to fatigue and low-back pain. This is followed by increased rates of diabetes, heart disease, cancer and other diseases. Dysfunction and disease are, in large part, due to not taking care of the body.

Since most of us have lost the natural tendency to be active like our very recent ancestors, we must satisfy that need artificially, by exercising. Without some fitness activity, you can't improve your level of health. And don't forget the issue of balance; too much activity can also impair your health.

Steps to improving your health may include eating real foods rather than processed, obtaining real vitamins and other nutrients from foods rather than synthetic vitamin supplements, and controlling stress. These and other specifics are discussed throughout this book.

With the realization that fitness and health are different also came the conclusion that these states are elements of an even larger concept — human performance. When health and fitness are balanced, the result is optimal human performance. We often associate human performance with the fulfillment of some athletic feat, like winning an Olympic gold medal. But in the true sense, human performance pertains to all aspects of life, including personal, family, social and work functions. Performance pertains to either physical or mental activities, or both. The benefits of improved human performance include increased energy, productivity, creativity, and better relationships with people. In my practice I had the pleasure and excitement to actually see people improve their human performance, and thus succeed at whatever their primary goal in life was at the time. These goals included winning the Ironman Triathlon, achieving career success, and being the best-possible parent. The secret to reaching any of these goals is optimal human performance, and its foundation is *balanced fitness and health*. Thus, we can define human performance as the optimal balance between health and fitness that allows a person to achieve success in all areas of life. Or, the simple equation:

Fitness + Health = Human Performance

This is a relatively simple concept to understand, but it's important to note that this equation is not one-directional, as its effects are actually cyclical and exponential. In other words, increased human performance can, in return, also bring about even greater improvements in the foundational elements of fitness and heath. Thus, as you improve your fitness and health, thereby improving your human performance, this additional human performance can fuel even further improvements in your fitness and health. There's virtually no end to this cycle, meaning that a person can achieve virtually unlimited physical and mental energy. It's really just a matter of how far you are willing to go to improve your fitness and your health.

2

Unlimited Physical and Mental Energy

The human body must produce large amounts of energy for all physical and mental activities. With proper balance between health and fitness, the body will have no trouble meeting the energy requirements for optimal human performance. But where does this energy come from? The answer is both simple and complex. Basically, energy comes from the sun. Light energy from the sun comes to earth and is converted to chemical energy in plants through the process of photosynthesis. We eat the plants, and most of us eat animals that eat plants. The chemical energy we take in is converted to mechanical energy that fuels all our physical and mental activities.

More directly, the energy produced by the body comes from the foods we eat. This energy is obtained from the basic macronutrients in food — carbohydrate, fat and protein. Though many foods contain all three, there's usually a predominance of one of these in each food. Consider the following examples:

- Carbohydrates are predominant in bread, sugar, rice, pasta, fruit and fruit juice, cereal.

- Fats are dominant in oil, butter, cheese, egg yolk.

- Protein is highest in meat, fish, poultry, eggs, cheese.

The majority of energy is produced from two of these food groups — carbohydrate and fat. Only a small amount, up to 15 percent of total energy, is produced from protein (by conversion of certain amino acids into glucose).

All three macronutrients are converted into energy in two steps. First, they are broken down in the intestine and absorbed into the blood as glucose from carbohydrates, fatty acids from fats, and amino acids from protein.

In the second step, the blood ultimately carries these elements to the cells, where the molecules of glucose, fatty acids and amino acids are further broken down. The hydrogen atom, the common building block of all three, is released as a result of further chemical breakdown. This atom contains one electron that is highly charged with energy. This electron is finally converted to a substance called ATP, which the body uses as energy.

So, to get more specific, we could say the body's energy comes from hydrogen's electron. Carbohydrates, fats and proteins each have different amounts of hydrogen molecules, and, therefore, potential energy. Fats have by far the most hydrogen, one reason we can get much more energy from the fats in food. Fats can actually provide more than twice the potential energy you get from either carbohydrates or protein.

Where does all this energy-generating activity take place? Mostly it is produced by your metabolism in the cells, especially in aerobic muscle fibers, which primarily use fat as a fuel. When these muscles are functioning optimally, you can derive even more energy from fat. In fact, up to 90 percent of your energy at any given time can come from fat, and the energy supply is virtually endless — the average lean person has enough stored fat to endure a 1,000-mile trek!

The more energy you derive from fat the better your fitness, health and human performance. By improving your fat-burning system, you'll improve metabolic efficiency and have more physical and mental energy. In addition, your body will store less fat, and you'll maintain a more stable blood-sugar level because you won't need as much sugar for energy.

When you don't produce the required amount of energy from fat, your body instead relies too heavily on sugar, usually producing fatigue. This common symptom, fatigue, is one of the most common complaints heard by doctors. It comes in physical and mental forms, or in a combination of both. Some people say they just can't perform as they did when they were younger. But age is no excuse for a lack of energy. Physical fatigue may strike at a particular time of the day, or it may make you feel exhausted from the time you awaken. You may feel you don't have the energy to do extra chores, go out at night or even get up in the morning. Mental fatigue is also common, making it difficult to think clearly or make decisions. This can affect anyone from students and executives to children and adults at all ages.

To avoid fatigue and instead access unlimited energy from your fat-burning system, two things must occur. First, you need to develop and utilize the body's aerobic system. Second, you need to provide that system with the proper fuel in the form of food. These items are discussed in the coming chapters.

To maintain efficient fat-burning, you also must burn some sugar. Herein lies another example of balance. Both fat and sugar are almost always being burned for energy at all times. It's a question of how much of each we use. Right now, you may be getting half of your energy from fat and half from sugar. When you improve your aerobic system and fat-burning capabilities, you may be able to obtain 70 percent of your energy from fat and 30 percent from sugar. But many people only get 10 percent of their energy from fat, forcing a full 90 percent to come from sugar. That's a very inefficient and unhealthy way to get energy. This is the typical situation in people who are fatigued and attempt to obtain more energy from sugar because they can't get much from fat. And when fat is not used for energy, it is stored in the body. This book explains how to reverse this situation and improve your fat-burning system.

This mix of fuels used for energy can be easily measured in a person, and is something I have done during my years in practice and during other research. So when I say you can improve your fat-burning capability, it is because I have seen and recorded these changes in actual patients. These measurements are taken using a gas analyzer, which measures the amount of oxygen a person inhales and the amount of carbon dioxide exhaled. The ratio of carbon dioxide to oxygen gives the percentage of fat and sugar that is used for energy. This is referred to as the respiratory quotient, or RQ. I usually don't recommend getting tested because for most people, when fat-burning is poor, there are plenty of signs and symptoms. These include the obvious — increased fat storage. Others include fatigue, blood sugar problems, hormone imbalance, poor circulation and even common physical injuries. Others are discussed throughout this book. In general, as fat-burning improves the body is able to correct many of its own problems. The bottom line — more fat-burning improves health, fitness and human performance.

3

Assessing Function
and Preventing Disease

We've now seen how balancing your health and fitness can lead to greater human performance, and provide for more energy for all aspects of your life. But more often than not, some piece of this equation gets out of balance. The result is some type of bodily dysfunction that, over time, can become some named disease. We're all too familiar with the common diseases, such as heart disease, cancer and stroke. But how do these diseases begin? The truth is most diseases don't just happen overnight. They have their beginnings as some relatively minor functional problem due to some imbalance of health and fitness. Reducing these problems in their earliest stages, which is relatively easy to do and a key focus of this book, is the best way to avoid disease. These seemingly innocent functional problems, often erroneously associated with aging, are termed functional illnesses.

Functional Illness

There are often no particular names for various early stages of disease development. There are simply signs and symptoms, and previous to that you may get no clues that a problem is arising. These signs and symptoms, as subtle as they may be, are known as functional problems, or functional illness. They are sometimes referred to as pre-disease, pre-clinical or, in the case of cancer, pre-malignant. Functional illness is that gray area between optimal health and disease.

Many people have some signs and symptoms of functional illness, such as fatigue, headaches, indigestion, back pain, allergies and dozens of other complaints. Not only can functional illness be the early stage of disease, it can also interfere with present quality of life. It's not normal to have these problems; it's a sign that something is wrong. The shelves of grocery stores and pharmacies are loaded with products made to medicate and mask these minor illnesses. But covering the problem does not make it go away, and worse yet, it turns off the body's attempt to tell you there's something wrong. These types of signs and symptoms aren't really addressed by mainstream medicine, which usually deals only with disease, the after-effect of functional illness.

Case History

John went to the company doctor for his annual physical examination. Many tests were performed — a very complete evaluation. The next week when John returned for the results, the doctor said, "Good news, everything looks great, there's nothing wrong." True, everything from blood pressure to cholesterol, clear lungs to strong heart was great news, but John was now more confused. He asked, "Then why do I have these headaches, and why is my energy so low? And why does my stomach always hurt after eating?" The doctor had no answer other than to say that he had ruled out disease.

In ruling out disease, John's doctor performed a vital service. But it was only the first step in evaluating John's fitness and health. Though John didn't have any disease, he had symptoms that made him uncomfortable and were interfering with his quality of life. What's more, these symptoms could be pointing to bigger problems down the road. This is a common example of functional illness.

Such functional illness — or dysfunction — is often the precursor to disease. By assessing your level of function you can find and correct many problems before they become diseases. As a clinician, a significant part of my initial examination of a patient was listening to his or her problems. I heard the main complaints of "I'm tired all day" or "my back hurts," but I more closely tuned in to other details such as waking in the middle of the night and being unable to get back to sleep, or exactly at what time of day the back felt worse, and when it was OK. Most of what I needed to know came from the patient telling me things of which he or she was not fully aware. These kinds of clues, the subtle and the obvious ones, and what they mean, are functional problems discussed throughout this book.

One way to know if you have a functional illness is through self-assessment. When we start listening to ourselves we will begin to get many clues. Once we have collected these clues, sorting them out becomes another art form. The most important distinction to make is the difference between primary and secondary problems. This is associated with what I call the domino effect.

The body tends to accumulate problems, often beginning with one small, seemingly minor imbalance. This problem causes another subtle imbalance, which triggers another, then several more. In the end, you get a symptom. It's like lining up a series of dominoes. All you need to do is knock down the first one and many others will fall too. What caused the last one to fall? Obviously it wasn't the one before it, or the one before that, but the first one. The body works the same way. The initial problem is often unnoticed. It's not until some of the later "dominoes" fall that more obvious clues and symptoms appear. In the end, you get a headache, fatigue or depression — or even disease. When you try to treat the last domino — treat just the end-result symptom — the cause of the problem isn't addressed. The first domino is the cause, or primary problem, and is often asymptomatic, meaning that you don't notice it. The next dominoes are the main complaint, or secondary problem, which produces the symptom but is merely the result of the first domino. The final domino is disease itself. Being able to differentiate between primary and secondary problems is important for all of us, including health-care professionals. The classic example is treating a diseased organ. A heart-bypass operation or removing a cancerous growth satisfies the end result. But what about the cause of the problem? If it's not found, how long will it take before another major problem arises, if it hasn't already?

As you become more intuitive about your health, you will begin to understand the signs and symptoms your body is providing in its desire to get your attention and your help. Once you develop your instincts, you'll be able to take responsibility to care for your own health. For those who can't or won't assess for functional illness and take appropriate actions to correct problems, there's always disease.

Disease

We can define disease quite simply as a gross imbalance of normal body function. Disease is the end result of dysfunction, usually expressed by signs and symptoms, of something in the body that has gone wrong. Heart disease, for example, begins many years or decades before the first sign of its presence appears (the most common one, unfortunately, being death). For almost all diseases there's a buildup of imbalances, and this eventually causes the end-result diagnosable disease.

Perhaps the most important question you should ask yourself is: Are there indications of these diseases earlier, in the pre-disease state? The answer is most definitely, yes! Your body usually tells you when something is going out of balance. In the case of heart disease, for example, abnormal blood cholesterol ratios or chronic inflammation, as discussed in later chapters, could be indications you are at risk. Both can be assessed through simple blood tests. These signs of dysfunction may exist years before the disease. What about even before your cholesterol goes askew? It's well known that men who develop even moderate amounts of abdominal fat are at much higher risk for a heart attack. And, symptoms like sleepiness and intestinal bloating after meals begin long before the fat begins showing up on the abdomen. Even early clues such as being overfat in childhood, and even birth weight, may be predictive.

Diet and Genes

The maturing field of genetics is showing us what many clinicians have suspected for years — foods can immediately influence the genetic blueprint. This information helps us better understand that genes are under our control and not something we must obey.

Consider identical twins, both individuals are given the same genes. In mid-life, one twin develops cancer, and the other lives a long healthy life without cancer. A specific gene instructed one twin to develop cancer, but in the other the same gene did not initiate the disease. One possibility is that the healthy twin had a diet that turned off the cancer gene — the same gene that instructed the other person to get sick. For many years, scientists have recognized other environmental factors, such as chemical toxins (tobacco for example), can contribute to cancer through their actions on genes. The notion that food has a specific influence on gene expression is relatively new.

From the moment of conception, the genes our parents give us provide continuous molecular instructions to cells and tissues, and ultimately the heart, lungs, brain, muscles and the rest of the body. In doing so, your health is regulated by what would seem to be a predetermined set of plans. However, genes, along with their diverse set of detailed instructions, are significantly influenced by the very foods you eat, and at each meal. In fact, the whole process of aging — how well we age and how long we live — is controlled throughout our lives through the impact on genes by nutrition.

The foods we eat can actually turn on, or turn off specific genes, and with it, detailed instructions regarding specific diseases. The bottom line: A good diet turns off genes that cause disease, and a bad diet turns on disease-causing genes. While we all have genes for diseases, they act like a light switch — they can be turned on, or turned off. The diet is like a finger controlling the switch. So what you eat — the quality and quantity of food at each meal — can dictate whether you turn on a particular genetic switch for diabetes, for example. The same is true for virtually all the problems that reduce quality of life, and for the diseases that kill us. This also includes being overweight — whether your parents were overfat or not isn't the issue but rather how and what you eat.

Many people use "genetics" as an excuse for their health problems — "my parents had this problem," "my grandfather had that problem." This attempt to justify ill health is no longer valid. Unfortunately, this defense is propagated throughout our culture, with the media partly to blame. Headlines touting "research shows addiction is genetic" or "obesity gene discovered" is a distortion of the truth promoted to sell newspapers and magazines.

Let's look at the facts. We may be predisposed to addiction or obesity, predisposed to diabetes, heart disease, cancer or many other problems, but if we become addicted, fat, diabetic etc., we are to blame, not our genes.

Gene Exceptions

A handful of true genetic disorders are the exception to this rule, and are rare. These include damage or other unwanted changes to genetic materials that occur soon after fertilization (some of these changes may even be part of the "natural selection" process humans continue to experience). After fertilization when mom and dad's cells share their genetic materials and begin to divide, changes in the genetic code no longer occur. At this point, the information in the genes no longer changes. From that point on it's the diet that controls the genetic switches. Conditions not considered to have a strong dietary or other environmental influence on genes include Rh incompatibility, sickle cell anemia and hemophilia. In addition, genetic injury can occur anytime throughout life, such as with radiation damage. Even though so-called genetic diseases may exist in an individual, whether that disease is genetically expressed — and whether it is severe or mild, or not evident at all — may be mostly influenced by diet, and other environmental factors such as toxic exposures.

Foods that can dramatically affect our genes include high-glycemic carbohydrates, especially processed starches and other grains, and sugar — bread, bagels, cereals, muffins, potatoes, and sugar and sugar-containing products including all popular soft drinks. In addition to the poor nutritional value of these foods, they release specific hormones, such as insulin, that adversely affect the body's metabolism. These foods also trigger genetic switches, turning on diseases such as diabetes, cancer, Alzheimer's disease, heart disease and many others. A low-glycemic meal, one without refined flours and sugars, can switch off the genes for these diseases.

A recent study published in the *American Journal of Clinical Nutrition* (May 2007) demonstrated how a high-glycemic meal switches on the genes that increase stress and inflammation (conditions that pave the way for most chronic disease) while turning off the genes that promote health.

Currently, billions of dollars are being spent in hopes of developing new drugs that will "switch" our genes in a certain direction. However, we already have the power to control our genetics in a natural way with diet. And, we have the ability to control future generations as well. Consider, for example, a couple starting a family — if one or both parents switch off healthy genes or turn on unhealthy genes the children can be even more vulnerable to disease.

Assessing for these signs in order to prevent disease is an important aspect of maintaining your fitness, health and human performance. We'll discuss more specifics about assessing for functional problems and avoiding disease throughout life's journey, which I call the human race.

4
Welcome to the Human Race

Most people don't think of themselves as athletes or competitors. The fact is, we're all in a race: the human race. We run to work, rush through business, race through lunch, dash to the store and tear through our errands. As we get older, life seems to get more complicated rather than easier, and more time-consuming. We wonder how we'll keep up this pace for the rest of our lives. The truth is, most people don't. The average person spends the last dozen or more years of life in a state of gross dysfunction, relying on others for care and just waiting to die. Many spend a lifetime of savings to maintain a few more moments of a poor-quality life. Instead of enjoying the road to life's finish line, most people reach it only after an agonizing death march.

Welcome to the human race. It's analogous to a very long journey, say, of 1,000 miles. If you were going to go that distance, you'd have to prepare for it, following certain rules. You'd have to find the foods that best match your individual needs for optimal energy. It would require physical preparation. You would need to assess for dysfunction to prevent injury and disease. You would have to make lifestyle adjustments along the way that increase your fitness, health and human performance. If your life is like a 1,000-mile journey, just how are you preparing for it?

A healthy person has enough body fat to fuel a 1,000-mile journey. And, I've actually trained athletes who successfully completed long endurance races, including 1,000-mile ultramarathons, Ironman triathlons and others. And many, including Mark Allen and Colleen Cannon, continue to be successful following their careers as professional athletes. To achieve their athletic feats, their training wasn't excessive. In many ways, these athletes employed a basic program similar to the one you can use in your life's journey as discussed in this book.

The human race is a true test of endurance. We are all endurance animals, and must use the natural endurance we all possess by unlocking our aerobic and fat-burning systems through proper nutrition and conditioning. Most patients I've seen — athletes and non-athletes alike — initially had gross deficiencies in their endurance. They could not keep up in life's journey.

Endurance is fueled by the aerobic system, encompassing, in part, the heart, lungs, blood vessels and especially the aerobic muscle fibers. Here, the energy is provided by nutrients obtained from the right kinds of foods, including fats, and generated by aerobic activity. If you "turn on" this aerobic system with easy exercise and the right foods, you will burn more fat and perform well in the human race.

There's another system at work in the body, which burns mostly sugar: This is the anaerobic system used for short-term speed. This is what you use when sprinting for the train, or chasing after a toddler. It's also the system that revs up when you're under stress. Too much anaerobic activity will cause the body to burn more sugar, and reduce the burning of fat and even store it. This fat may accumulate in the blood vessels, abdomen or hips. Overuse of the anaerobic system will produce symptoms that may include mental and physical fatigue, moodiness, low blood sugar and recurrent or chronic injury, to name a few. And, it reduces your endurance. If you try to get through life's journey using this system, you're apt to have a very hard time.

Imbalances in the aerobic and anaerobic systems result from poor lifestyle habits, including under- and over-training, and are often instigated by popular but dangerous social trends and misinformation. Examples include "get fit quick" programs and fast weight-loss scams. We must all run our own race. Beyond the basic rules, everyone has individual requirements. Each of you can discover your own needs for a personal best in life's journey.

If you try to run life's race in a random way, things won't go well. But if you're properly prepared for life's long journey, you can achieve a world-class performance. This is a book about preparing for life's journey.

In the following chapters I'll discuss specifics of food and nutrition, physical activity and self-health management that can help you succeed in the human race. I hope to see you at the finish line.

5

Choose Your Food Wisely

All animals on earth know how to eat. However, most humans have lost their instinctive ability to make wise food choices and instead look elsewhere for advice. Unfortunately, we are inundated with messages about how and what to eat — mostly from unreliable sources.

Food is the foundation of everything you do. Without the right fuel for the aerobic system, fat-burning will be limited. Without the thousands of nutrients from food, the immune system can't stop the process of disease. And without the necessary balance of macronutrients, the brain can't continue to thrive.

In order to achieve optimal human performance, wise decisions about the foods you eat are essential. The best foods help the body produce nearly unlimited energy, increase fat-burning and lead to a healthy life. In addition, the body is constantly making new cells, and, in fact, always replacing itself, so you're really making a new body all the time. The building blocks for this new body come from the foods you eat. So, in a very real sense, you really are what you eat.

Just as each of us has a different set of fingerprints, the specific requirements for carbohydrates, fats and proteins, along with the right amounts of vitamins, minerals and fiber, can vary from person to person. To build and maintain optimal health you must supply your body with the right mix of fuels and nutrients that matches your individual needs. This is much easier than you think, and what you'll learn in this book.

Unfortunately, many people obtain information about food and nutrition, and other key lifestyle issues as well, through newspapers, magazines, radio and TV. With few exceptions, this information is usually misguided — packaged and processed junk food disguised as healthy is continuously pushed on the public. While these sources may be entertaining, they're usually not an accurate source of health information. The goal of these media sources is to sell newspapers and magazines, and keep you listening or watching a certain program. One reason for the slanted information is the editorial process — many articles, interviews and other bits of information never get reported because the information clashes with advertisers. But in addition to their ads, these same advertisers get their information to the public in the form of articles, interviews and other media — even through sponsored "scientific studies" — often with the public not suspecting there's a conflict of interest.

There is a lot of money behind this campaign to sell you unhealthy food. Large corporations spend billions of dollars telling us to be hungry for unhealthy foods. And it works — how many times have you seen a commercial on TV and suddenly had an intense craving for whatever was being advertised? And how often did you feel the need to buy a certain product because the announcer or writer said it was the best thing for your health? The answer to both questions is *often* — that's the power of advertising and the way the media is intricately connected with advertisers.

Likewise, we cannot rely on the government to make our menu. Over the years and decades, the United States Department of Agriculture (USDA) has come up with many different recommendations — I often referred to these as pyramid schemes. While these are often associated with updates in scientific information, there is a heavy dose of special interest groups and lobbyists behind the recommendations. These include lobbyists for the dairy industry, from companies that make breakfast cereals and from those who have directly contributed to our current obesity epidemic — the sugar industry. From the old four food groups to the many changing pyramids, these recommendations include many unhealthy foods, such as refined carbohydrates and sugar, but have de-emphasized fresh vegetables and fruits. The best recommendation is for each of us to know our own food needs.

The truth is each person has his or her own food pyramid because we're all unique with individual requirements. However, there are some basic recommendations that may be helpful, and these will be emphasized throughout the book. These are the foundations of a food plan to build and maintain optimal human performance. The first is to only eat real food — not processed, not artificial, but foods provided by nature. Instead, common recommendations and the largest component of most people's diet include refined foods, especially carbohydrates — cereal, bread, bagels, rolls and rice — and sugar and sugar-containing foods. Another key feature of a healthy food plan is balancing fats by eating sufficient amounts of good fats and avoiding all bad fats. In addition, we all need moderate amounts of high quality protein. And, we all require sufficient amounts of fresh vegetables and fruits. We also need adequate amounts of pure water, something many people fail to achieve.

What's the basic recipe? Choose your food wisely.

6

The Carbohydrate Trend

As companies began refining healthy foods, making them sweeter and increasing shelf life, sometimes to months and years, the nutritional quality of these foods diminished significantly. This is true of carbohydrate foods more than any other. This includes the mass production of sugar that has grown dramatically as its use in many foods continues to increase. The result is that over the past few generations most people consume too much carbohydrate. Today, one obvious result is that overfat people now make up the majority! One reason is the fact that a significant portion of carbohydrate foods turns to fat in the body.

The trend in carbohydrate overconsumption continues today, propelled by companies selling refined carbohydrates and sugar. They've been so successful that the newest epidemic includes obese babies. This is due to the promotion of highly refined baby cereals, which are actually worse for babies than pure sugar.

For many generations, the common recommendations have been to eat a large amount of carbohydrates. And, if you've followed the USDA food pyramids through the years most of your diet is carbohydrate, and you've gotten fat. The problem goes beyond being fat — highly refined carbohydrate diets are unhealthy on all levels, significantly reducing human performance. Today, the term "carbohydrate" is almost always synonymous with "refined carbohydrate."

One reason for this imbalance is that the human body has not adapted to processing this amount of carbohydrates, especially in refined forms. For 99.6 percent of our existence on earth, humans consumed diets that were relatively low in almost all carbohydrates but higher in fat, protein and vegetables. During most of evolutionary history, humans lived near the sea and consumed significant amounts of fish, seafood, and other land-animal proteins. More importantly, significant amounts of plant foods were also consumed. These included vegetables, fruits, nuts and seeds, which help protect against the potential effects of high intakes of saturated fat. In addition, our ancestors were very active physically. Only in the last 5,000 years has this changed. The Agricultural Revolution brought a dramatic increase in carbohydrate foods, and the Industrial Revolution brought highly refined carbohydrates to the table. The intake of carbohydrates by humans has never been so dramatically high as it has been in just the last 100 years. This relatively short period of significant dietary change has contributed to many problems leading to heart disease, cancer, obesity and other diseases.

For most people, eating such a high-carbohydrate diet can reduce fat-burning and energy production, increase body-fat storage, significantly reduce overall health, and greatly diminish human performance.

Carbohydrates and Insulin

Common foods including breads and other items made with flour such as rolls, muffins, pancakes, waffles, cereals and pasta are among the highest in carbohydrates. Also included in this category are all sweets, including the hidden sugars found in many foods. One of the main problems associated with eating carbohydrates has to do with insulin.

Insulin is a hormone made by the pancreas. When you eat carbohydrate foods, they are digested and the carbohydrate is absorbed into the blood as glucose (blood sugar). This stimulates the release of insulin, which has many different jobs. Three key actions of insulin on blood sugar include the following:

- About 50 percent of the carbohydrate you eat is quickly used for energy in the body's cells. (Earlier we talked about getting energy from both sugar and fat — this is the part that comes from sugar.)

- About 10 percent of the carbohydrate you eat is converted to and stored as glycogen, a reserved form of sugar. When blood sugar is low, glycogen stored in the muscles and liver is converted back to glucose and used for energy. (Muscle glycogen is used for energy by the muscles containing it, and liver glycogen is used mostly to maintain blood-sugar levels between meals and during nighttime sleep.)

- About 40 percent of the carbohydrate you eat is converted to fat and stored.

Insulin production occurs as a normal process each and every time you eat a meal containing carbohydrates. Small amounts of insulin may also be produced if you consume a protein-only meal, and in some people, a high-protein meal can stimulate significant amounts of insulin. But for most people, it's predominantly carbohydrates that trigger the insulin mechanism.

The more carbohydrates consumed, the more insulin produced. For many people — especially those who are overfat and those who have consumed a high carbohydrate diet for a long time — eating carbohydrates results in production of too much insulin. This leads to a condition referred to as insulin resistance, and it's associated with the inability of insulin to efficiently fuel the cells, especially the muscle cells, with glucose. As a result, the cells do not get all the glucose they need for energy. When these people eat carbohydrates, the brain can get the message that the cells don't have enough sugar and it tells the pancreas to make more insulin. Finally, insulin is produced beyond normal limits, a condition referred to as hyperinsulinism — too much insulin. While it takes more insulin to get glucose into the insulin-resistant cells efficiently, this hormone still performs its other tasks, including converting carbohydrates to fat. As mentioned previously, in a normal person, 40 percent of the carbohydrates eaten is converted to fat. In a person who produces too much insulin, that number may be much higher, perhaps 50 to 60 percent.

In many people, this excess production of insulin may be amplified due to genetics, or it may be a normal response to eating too much carbohydrate. If you have a family history of diabetes, heart disease, high blood pressure or stroke, the odds are greater that you have less tolerance for carbohydrate consumption. Lifestyle also contributes to this problem, including poor dietary habits such as eating too much carbohydrate, too little protein, lack of exercise and stress.

But even if diabetes runs in your family, you still may be able to control the problem with the proper lifestyle factors.

In addition to causing even more carbohydrates to convert and store as fat, excess insulin can lower the blood sugar too drastically. Since the brain exclusively relies on glucose for fuel, this can result in impaired mental function, including loss of memory, reduced concentration and other cognitive function. Low blood sugar also often results in hunger, sometimes only a couple of hours, or less, after the meal. Cravings, often for sweets, are frequently part of this cycle, and resorting to snacking on more carbohydrates maintains the cycle. And if you don't eat, you just feel worse. Eventually, the fat-storage deposits get bigger.

High insulin levels also suppress two important hormones: glucagon and growth hormone. Glucagon has the opposite effect of insulin and is produced following protein consumption. While insulin promotes storage, glucagon promotes the utilization of fat and sugar for energy. Growth hormone is also important for sugar- and fat-burning, the regulation of minerals, and amino-acid action on muscle development.

If your goal is to burn more body fat, improve your health and increase human performance, you must eliminate refined carbohydrates, and determine how much natural carbohydrate your body can effectively metabolize. This will vary from person to person. Before discussing how that is accomplished, let's look at some other important aspects of carbohydrates and insulin.

Measuring the Insulin Response

The glycemic index (GI) is an indicator of how much your blood sugar increases after eating specific carbohydrate foods. However, it must be noted that glycemic index is only a very general measure of responses to food, and individual variation is not considered in studies of foods and their glycemic effects. High-GI foods, which produce the greatest glucose response, include bagels, breads, potatoes, sweets and other foods that contain refined flour and sugar. Many processed cereals, especially those containing the sugar maltose, which has a very high GI, produce an even stronger glucose response. Even foods you may think are good for you can trigger high amounts of insulin, including fruit juice and bananas. The biggest problems in most diets may be wheat products, potatoes, fruit juice and sugar or sugar-containing products.

Carbohydrates with a lower GI include some fruits, such as grapefruits and cherries, and legumes such as lentils. Non-carbohydrate foods, proteins and fats, usually don't cause a glycemic problem, although in some people even meals high in protein and/or fat can trigger an abnormal insulin response. In these situations, eating smaller and more frequent low-glycemic meals often solves the problem, as discussed later.

Most vegetables contain only small amounts of carbohydrates (except very starchy ones like potatoes and corn). Carrots were at one time believed to be a high-glycemic food, but studies have shown the glycemic effect of this root vegetable to be relatively low.

Insulin responses to carbohydrate intake and the ensuing blood-sugar rise can vary greatly from person to person. But generally, more refined carbohydrates evoke a stronger and more rapid production of insulin. One reason for this, as discussed earlier, is that humans are not adapted to diets high in carbohydrates, so our metabolism is not meant to process these foods. Another reason is that refined carbohydrates lack the natural fiber that helps moderate the carbohydrate/glucose and insulin responses. Consumption of natural fiber with carbohydrates can reduce the dietary stress associated with high-carbohydrate meals.

In practical terms, this means that eating refined foods like a cookie or piece of cake will cause more problems than eating a piece of fruit or whole-grain crackers with the same amount of carbohydrate and calories. Low-fat foods or low-fat meals containing carbohydrates have a relatively higher glycemic index. This is due to quicker digestion and absorption of sugar when less fat is present.

Eating carbohydrate foods in combination with some fats, such as olive oil or butter, slows digestion and absorption, thus moderating the insulin response. Moderate protein levels in a meal also can lower the glycemic index of the meal. Artificial sweeteners should also be avoided as even these foods can trick the brain and cause insulin responses through what is known as the cephalic phase of digestion.

By moderating carbohydrate intake to control insulin production, you can increase your ability to burn fat as an optimal and efficient source of almost unlimited energy. Rather than using the glycemic index as a guide, which has become more common, especially among diabetics, all individuals should learn which foods and food combinations work best for their individual needs. This is most easily accomplished by performing the Two-Week Test, along with proper follow-up, as discussed in the next chapter.

Carbohydrate Intolerance

With generations of people over-consuming carbohydrates, many now have a problem I call carbohydrate intolerance, or CI. It's now an epidemic. CI begins as a functional problem that negatively affects quality of life and gradually results in serious illness and disease. Though most people are unaware such a condition even exists in its early stages, a high percentage of the population suffers from CI in its early and later stages. The symptoms of early CI are very common and include sleepiness after meals, intestinal bloating, increased body fat, fatigue and many others listed in the survey that follows.

CI is referred to by other names, but it is best viewed as one long progression of the same problem. In the early stages, the symptoms can be elusive, often associated with blood-sugar problems, fatigue, intestinal bloating and loss of concentration. In the middle stages, the worsening condition may be referred to as carbohydrate-lipid metabolism disturbance, and cause more serious conditions such as hypertension, elevations of LDL and lowering of HDL cholesterol, elevated triglycerides, excess body fat and often obesity. In the long term, CI manifests itself as various diseases, including diabetes, cancer and heart disease. These end-stage conditions are part of a set of diseases now well recognized and referred to as Syndrome X, or the Metabolic Syndrome. To make this process easy to understand, the full spectrum of these problems can simply be referred to as CI.

Young people with CI are at much higher risk for disease later in life. For example, those with CI have an estimated tenfold greater risk for developing diseases such as diabetes. Some individuals who ultimately become diabetic display symptoms of carbohydrate intolerance 20 years or more before the onset of disease. Even birth weight can be a predictor of CI.

Like many problems, CI is an individual one, affecting different people in different ways. Only you can determine how intolerant you are to carbohydrates, and to what degree. Blood tests will diagnose the problem only in the middle and latter stages, but the symptoms may have begun years earlier. The key to avoiding the full spectrum of CI is to be aware of it in its earliest stage, and to make the appropriate diet and lifestyle changes. This will improve quality of life immediately and prevent the onset of disease later. However, for those already in a disease state, significant immediate improvements can still be made with the proper adjustments.

Following is a list of some common complaints of people with CI. Many occur immediately following a carbohydrate meal, and others are constant. While keeping in mind that these signs and symptoms may also be related to other causes, ask yourself if you have any of these problems:

❑ **Physical fatigue.** Whether you call it fatigue or exhaustion, the most common feature of CI is that it wears people out. Some are tired just in the morning or afternoon; others are exhausted all day.

❑ **Mental fatigue.** Sometimes the fatigue of CI is physical, but often it's mental (as opposed to psychological); the inability to concentrate is the most evident symptom. Loss of creativity, poor memory, and failing or poor grades in school often accompany CI, as do various forms of "learning disabilities." This is much more pronounced immediately after a meal, or if a meal is delayed or missed. The worker who returns to his or her job site after lunch, only to be unable to concentrate due to mental fatigue, is a very common example. Some actually fall asleep at their desk after lunch.

❑ **Blood-sugar problems.** The blood sugar may be normal until a carbohydrate meal is consumed, or if meals are not eaten on a regular schedule. Periods of erratic blood sugar, including abnormal hypoglycemia, accompanied by many of the symptoms listed here, are not normal. Feeling jittery, agitated and moody is common with CI, and is relieved almost immediately once food is eaten. Dizziness is also common, as is the craving for sweets, chocolate or caffeine. These symptoms are not necessarily associated with abnormal blood-sugar levels, but may be related to neurological stress, possibly due to the changes in blood sugar and insulin.

❏ **Intestinal bloating.** Foods that produce the most intestinal gas are complex carbohydrates, specifically starches, such as wheat products and potatoes, and other non-starch carbohydrates such as sugar. People with CI often suffer from excessive gas production. Antacids, or other remedies for symptomatic relief, are not very successful in dealing with the problem. The gas tends to build and is worse later in the day and at night.

❏ **Sleepiness.** Many people with CI get sleepy immediately after meals containing more than their limit of carbohydrates. This is typically a pasta meal, or even a meat meal that includes bread, potatoes or dessert.

❏ **Increased body fat.** For most people, too much weight is too much fat. In males, an increase in abdominal fat is more evident and an early sign of CI (I call this the "carbo belly"). In females, it's more prominent in the upper body compared to the thighs and legs. In the face, "chipmunk cheeks" may be a telltale sign.

❏ **Increased triglycerides.** High triglycerides in the blood are often seen in people with CI. These triglycerides are the direct result of dietary carbohydrates being converted by insulin into fat. In my experience, fasting triglyceride levels over 100 mg/dl may be an indication of a carbohydrate-intolerance problem (even though 100 is in the so-called normal range).

❏ **High blood pressure.** Most people with hypertension have CI. There is often a direct relationship between insulin levels and blood pressure — as average insulin levels elevate, so does blood pressure. For some, regardless of whether the blood pressure is elevated, sodium sensitivity is common and eating too much sodium causes water retention along with elevated blood pressure.

❑ **Depression.** Because carbohydrates can be a natural "downer," depression is common among people who have CI. Carbohydrates do this by adversely affecting levels of neurotransmitters made in the brain, producing feelings of depression. Many people have been taught that sugar is stimulating, but actually the opposite can be true. Some people have a short, initial burst of energy after eating sugar, but it does not last. This is a significant consideration for children or adults trying to function optimally at school, home or work.

In addition to the signs and symptoms listed above, carbohydrates, especially sugar, can be addicting. Some people have trouble accepting that notion as there are no clear scientific studies to demonstrate the claim. Many professionals have struggled trying to help patients who could not reduce or eliminate sugar despite its unhealthy hold on them.

We still don't have a clear scientific study that shows sugar or other refined carbohydrate foods can be addicting. However, some studies do show that certain foods, like sugar, can trigger the brain's reward centers — the same brain areas stimulated by cocaine, nicotine and other well-accepted addicting substances.

The fact that food can be addicting is well accepted — and even proven — by the very companies who use addiction as a powerful tool to sell these products. Food advertisers, who spend billions of dollars each year, know very well about addiction, and how to tease you with foods that can kill you. These ad campaigns are especially successful with children, and they are not unlike those used by the tobacco industry for so many decades.

If society placed sugar in the same category as cigarettes, there would be a revolution. State, city and even federal government agencies would ban sugar and refined carbohydrate foods due to the astronomical cost of health care associated with its addiction. Companies that make cereals, candies, cookies and sugar itself would be sued, much like the tobacco class-action lawsuits of recent history. I can imagine the secret after-school cookie deals, sugar at $650 a pound, or by prescription only, and the growth of sugar addiction clinics where the treatment of choice would be artificial sweeteners. Well, things may be heading that way.

With some countries banning sugar food ads on children's TV, banning of soda in schools, restaurants being required to post calories in their meals, and other restrictions, the war has begun. Science is catching up too. But let's not rely on the government, science or anything or anyone else to get us to act. Like other addictions we are the responsible parties. There is help if we need it, but after a long time in clinical practice it's clear to me that each of us holds the key to control or eliminate (depending on the definitions) addiction despite the ongoing propaganda from big corporations who continue to peddle their deadly foods.

Not only can carbohydrates be addictive, but CI is a prevalent problem in persons addicted to alcohol, caffeine, cigarettes or other drugs. Often, the drug is the secondary problem, with CI being the primary one. Treating this primary problem should obviously be a major focus of any addiction therapy, which can make recovering from other drugs more successful.

Other groups of people are very vulnerable to CI, including those who are inactive, under stress, taking estrogen, dark skinned and those with a family history of diabetes and other diseases of the metabolic syndrome. In addition, aging is frequently accompanied by increased carbohydrate intolerance.

The Metabolic Syndrome

If CI is not corrected in the early stages, your signs and symptoms, and your overall health can easily worsen and even lead to disease. There is a whole complex of related diseases that include some of the biggest killers of today: heart disease, cancer, stroke, diabetes and others. These diseases kill more people in the United States each year than died in all of our wars combined. This disease complex is referred to as the Metabolic Syndrome (or Syndrome X). The specific disorders include:

- Hyperinsulinemia

- Diabetes (type 2)

- Hypertension

- Obesity

- Polycystic ovary

- Stroke

- Breast cancer

- Coronary heart disease

- Hyperlipidemia (high blood cholesterol and triglycerides)

These problems don't necessarily all develop or even evolve in this order. But all are related to CI. Unfortunately, once some of these diseases develop, many of the changes are more difficult to treat conservatively, and more extreme care may be needed. However, even these conditions can improve with the right dietary control, which includes solving the problem of excess carbohydrate intake.

How do you adjust your lifestyle so that carbohydrate intolerance is not a problem? Before you do anything, you need to know just how sensitive you are to carbohydrates. Your doctor may do some tests, including checking insulin and glucose levels, to see if the problem can be detected. You could just follow a low-carbohydrate diet, but the better choice is to determine your own specific needs.

Finding your optimal level of carbohydrate intake is the first step to balancing the rest of your diet. In the mid 1980s I developed an effective method of finding the optimal level of carbohydrate intake. It's called the Two-Week Test and is detailed in the following chapter.

7

The Two-Week Test

If you have some or all the signs and symptoms of carbohydrate intolerance, the next step is to evaluate how your body functions without high amounts of carbohydrates. The Two Week Test begins with a period of time in which your insulin levels are moderated because your carbohydrate intake is decreased. Based on your signs and symptoms, this can help determine if you are carbohydrate intolerant, and if so, how to remedy it. I must emphasize that this is only a test, and it will only last two weeks — you will not be eating like this forever. And most importantly, this is not a diet. You should not be hungry as you can eat as much of the non-carbohydrate foods as you want, and as often as you need.

I developed the Two-Week Test almost 25 years ago. Thousands of people have used it to get healthy, lose body fat and significantly improve human performance. Others have found it the best way to jumpstart their metabolism because it quickly shifts the body into a high fat-burning state. Still others have reduced or eliminated medications they once required. For many, it has turned their lives around. Of all the tools I've used through my career, the Two Week Test continues to surprise me — at how a person can go from one extreme of poor health to great health in such a short time. It's simply a matter of removing a major stress in a person's life and allowing the body to heal and function at a very healthy level.

It is not the purpose of the test to restrict calories or fat. It merely restricts moderate- and high-glycemic carbohydrates. Nor is its purpose to avoid all carbohydrates, or go into ketosis like other diet regimes. And, there's no need to weigh food or count grams or calories. Just eat what you're allowed, and avoid what should be avoided for two weeks.

Let's discuss all the aspects of the Two Week Test, and at the end of the chapter I'll summarize them so you have a concise list to follow.

Before you start the test, ask yourself about the signs and symptoms of carbohydrate intolerance described in the previous chapter. Write down the problems that you have from this list, along with any and all other complaints you have. This may take you a few days as many people are so used to certain problems they can't recall them all at once. This is very important because after the test, you will review these complaints to see which ones have improved.

Next, weigh yourself before starting the test. This is the only instance I recommend using the scale. During the test you may lose some excess water your body is holding, but you'll also go into a high fat-burning state and lose body fat. I've seen some people lose only a few pounds during the test, and some 20 or more pounds. This is not a weight-loss regime, and the main purpose of weighing yourself is to have another sign of how your body is working, especially after the test.

Before you start the test, make sure you have enough of the foods you'll be eating during the test — these are listed later in the chapter. Go shopping and stock up on these items. This requires a little planning, so make a list of the foods you want to eat and the meals and snacks you want to make available. In addition, go through your cabinets and refrigerator and get rid of any sweets in your house, or you'll be tempted. Remember, many people are addicted to sugar and other carbohydrates, and for the first few days you may crave these foods.

Planning is very important. Make sure you do not go hungry during the test! Schedule the test during a two-week period that you are relatively unlikely to have distractions — the holidays or times when social engagements are planned can make it too easy to stray from the plan. There are many foods to select from so you don't ever need to go hungry. Eat as much of the allowable foods as you want — there are many of them. Don't worry about cholesterol, fat or calories, or the amount of food you're eating. This is only a test, not the way you'll be eating all the time.

Plan to eat as much as you need to never be hungry. This means planning your meals and having snacks available. Most importantly, eat breakfast within an hour of waking.

Following the diet for less than two weeks probably will not give you a valid result. So, if after five days, for example, you eat a bowl of pasta or a box of cookies, you will need to start the test over.

Foods to Eat During the Test

You are allowed to eat as much of these foods as you like during the Two-Week Test:

- ✔ Eggs (whites and yolk), unprocessed (real) cheeses, heavy (whipping) cream, sour cream.
- ✔ Unprocessed meats including beef, turkey, chicken, lamb, fish, shellfish and others.
- ✔ Tomato, V-8 or other vegetable juices such as carrot juice.
- ✔ Water.
- ✔ Cooked or raw vegetables except potatoes and corn.
- ✔ Nuts, seeds, nut butters.
- ✔ Oils, vinegar, mayonnaise, salsa, mustard and spices.
- ✔ Sea salt, unless you are sodium sensitive.
- ✔ All coffee and tea (if you normally drink it).

Be sure to read the ingredients for many of these foods if they are packaged, as some form of sugar is commonly added.

Foods to Avoid During the Test

You may not eat the following foods during the Two-Week Test:

- ◌ Bread, rolls, pasta, pancakes, cereal, muffins, chips, crackers, rice cakes and similar carbohydrate foods.
- ◌ Sweets, including products that contain sugar such as ketchup, honey, and many other prepared foods (read the labels).
- ◌ Fruits and fruit juice.
- ◌ Highly processed meats such cold cuts, which often contain sugar.
- ◌ Potatoes (all types), corn, rice and beans.
- ◌ Milk, half-and-half and yogurt.
- ◌ So-called healthy snacks, including all energy bars and drinks.
- ◌ All soda, including so-called diet types.

A Note on Alcohol

If you normally drink small to moderate amounts of alcohol, some forms are allowed during the test.

Alcohol allowed: dry wines, and pure distilled spirits (gin, vodka, whiskey, etc.), and those mixed with plain carbonated water, including seltzer.

Alcohol not allowed: Sweet wines, all beer, Champaign, alcohol containing sugar (rum, liqueurs, etc.), and those mixed with sweet ingredients such as tonic, soda or other sugary liquids. If in doubt, avoid it.

Helpful Suggestions

Below are some other suggestions for eating, food preparation and dining out which may be helpful during the Two-Week Test. You may find these suggestions helpful after completing the test as well.

Meal Ideas

Eggs

- Omelets, with any combination of vegetables, meats and cheeses.
- Scrambled with guacamole, sour cream and salsa.
- Scrambled with a scoop of ricotta cheese and tomato sauce.
- Boiled or poached with spinach or asparagus and hollandaise or cheese sauce.
- With bacon or other meats.
- Soufflés.

Salads

- Chef — leaf lettuce, meats, cheeses, eggs.
- Spinach — with bacon, eggs, anchovies.
- Caesar — Romaine lettuce, eggs, Parmesan cheese, anchovies.
- Any salad with chicken, tuna, shrimp or other meat or cheese.

Salad Dressings

- Extra-virgin olive oil and vinegar (balsamic, wine, apple cider). Plain or with sea salt and spices.
- Creamy — made with heavy cream, mayonnaise, garlic and spices.

Fish and Meats

- Pot roast cooked with onions, carrots and celery.
- Roasted chicken stuffed with a bulb of anise, celery and carrots.
- Chili-type dish made with fresh, chopped meat and a variety of vegetables such as diced eggplant, onions, celery, peppers, zucchini, tomatoes and spices (no beans).
- Steak and eggs.
- Any meat with a vegetable and a mixed salad.
- Chicken parmigiana (not breaded or deep-fried) with a mixed salad.
- Fish (not breaded or deep-fried) with any variety of sauces and vegetables.
- Tuna melt on a bed of broccoli or asparagus.

Sauces

- Plain melted butter.
- A quick cream sauce can be made by simmering heavy cream with mustard or curry powder and cayenne pepper, or any flavor of choice. It's delicious over eggs, poultry and vegetables.
- Italian-style tomato sauce helps make a quick parmigiana out of any fish, meat or vegetables. Put this over spaghetti squash for a pasta-like dish. Or make lasagna with sliced grilled eggplant or zucchini instead of pasta.

Snacks

- Hard-boiled eggs.
- Slices of fresh meat and/or cheese wrapped in lettuce.

- Vegetable juices.
- Almonds, cashews, pecans.
- Celery stuffed with nut butter or cream cheese.
- Guacamole with vegetable sticks for dipping.
- Leftovers from a previous meal.

Dining Out
- Let the waiter know you do not want any bread, to avoid temptation.
- Ask for an extra vegetable instead of rice or potato.
- Chinese: Steamed meat, fish or vegetables (no rice or sweet sauce).
- Continental: steak, roast beef, duck, fish or seafood.
- French: Coquille Saint-Jacques, boeuf a la Bourguignonne.
- Italian: Veal parmigiana (not breaded or deep-fried), seafood marinara.
- Avoid all fried food as it usually has breading or is coated in flour.

After the Test
Re-evaluate your original list of complaints after the Two-Week Test. Is your energy better? Are you sleeping better? Less depressed? If you feel better now than you did two weeks ago, or if you lost weight, you probably have some degree of CI, and you're unable to eat as much carbohydrate as you did before the test. Some people who have a high degree of CI will feel dramatically better than they did before the test, especially if there was a large weight loss. Some people say they feel like a new person after taking this test. Others say after a few days of the test, they feel young again.

Check your weight. Any weight loss during the test is not due to reduced calories, as many people eat more calories than usual during this two-week period. It's due to the increased fat-burning resulting from reduced insulin. While there may be some water loss, especially if you are sodium sensitive, there is real fat loss.

If your blood pressure has been high, and especially if you are on medication, ask your health-care professional to check it several times during the test, and especially right after the test. Sometimes blood pressure drops significantly and your medication may need to be adjusted, or eliminated, which should only be done by your health-care professional. For many people, as insulin levels are reduced to normal, blood pressure normalizes too.

Finding Your Carbohydrate Tolerance

If nothing improved during the test — and it was done exactly as described above — then you may not be carbohydrate intolerant. But if the Two-Week Test improved your signs and symptoms, the next step is to determine how much carbohydrate you can tolerate, without a return of these problems. This is done by adding a single-serving size of natural unprocessed carbohydrates to every other meal or snack. The purpose is to determine if any of these carbohydrates cause the return of any of the original signs or symptoms, including weight gain, or even new problems. At this stage, having just completed the test, your body and brain will be more aware of even slight reactions to carbohydrate foods — basically, you'll be more intuitive to how your body responds to food. This is done in the following manner over the next one to two weeks:

Begin adding single-serving amounts of natural, unprocessed carbohydrates at every other meal or snack. This may be plain yogurt sweetened with a little honey for breakfast, or an apple after lunch or dinner. For a snack, try tea with honey or a healthy homemade energy bar (see the Phil's bar recipe). Avoid all refined carbohydrates such as sugar and refined-flour products (like white bread, cereals, rolls or pasta). In addition to fresh fruit, plain yogurt and honey, other suggestions include brown rice, sweet potatoes, yams, lentils and beans.

Most bread, crackers, cereals and other grains are processed and should be avoided — even those stating "whole grain" or "100% whole wheat." Read the ingredients carefully. If you can find real-food whole grain products, they can be used. These include sprouted breads, whole oats (they take 30-45 minutes to cook) and other dense products made with just ground wheat, rye or other grains. If in doubt, avoid them during this one- to two-week period.

I want to emphasize again not to add a carbohydrate in back-to-back meals or snacks, as insulin production is partly influenced by your previous meal.

With the addition of each carbohydrate, be aware of any symptoms you had previously that were eliminated by the test, especially symptoms that develop immediately after eating, such as intestinal bloating, sleepiness or feelings of depression.

Most importantly, if any signs or symptoms that disappeared during or following the Two Week Test have now returned, you've probably exceeded your carbohydrate limit. For example, if your hunger or cravings were greatly improved at the end of the test, and now they've returned, you probably added too many carbohydrates. If you lost eight pounds during the test, and gained back five pounds after adding some carbohydrates for a week or two, you've probably eaten too many carbohydrates. Likewise, if blood pressure rises significantly after it was reduced, it may be due to excess carbohydrate intake. If any of these situations occur, reduce the carbohydrates by half, or otherwise experiment to see which particular foods cause symptoms and which don't. Some people return to the Two Week Test and begin the process again.

In some cases, people can tolerate simple carbohydrates, such as fresh fruits, plain yogurt and honey, but not complex carbohydrates such as sweet potato, whole grains, beans or other starches. In other situations, some individuals don't tolerate any wheat products. During this post-test period, these factors are often easy to determine.

After this one- to two-week period of experimenting with natural carbohydrates, you'll have a very good idea about your body's level of carbohydrate tolerance. You'll better know which foods to avoid, which ones you can eat and those that must be limited. You'll become acutely aware of how your body feels when you eat too many carbohydrates. From time to time, you may feel the need to go through a Two-Week Test period again to check yourself, or to quickly get back on track after careless eating during the holidays, vacations or at other times.

Many people find the loss of grains in the diet leaves the digestive tract sluggish and a little constipated. After years of eating lots of carbohydrates, your intestine gets used to that type of bulk. If you become constipated during the Two-Week Test, or afterwards when a lower amount of carbohydrate in the diet is maintained, it could be due to a number of reasons. First, you may not be eating enough fiber (this topic is discussed in more detail in a later chapter). Bread, pasta and cereals are significant sources of fiber for many people.

Psyllium is a high-fiber herb that is a very effective promoter of intestinal function. Adding plain unsweetened psyllium to a glass of water, tomato juice or healthy smoothie can keep your system running smoothly — start with one teaspoon a day for a few days to make sure it's tolerated, then use up to about one tablespoon a day. Another way to add psyllium to your diet is to use it in place of flour for thickening sauces or in place of bread crumbs to coat meats and vegetables. If you require a fiber supplement, be sure to use the ones that do not contain sugar, so read the labels. There are some sugar-free psyllium products on the market and you should not have trouble finding one.

Another reason for constipation at this time may be dehydration. If you don't drink enough water, you could be predisposed to constipation. During the Two-Week Test, you'll need more water — up to two to three quarts or more per day. After the test, vegetables, legumes, such as lentils, and fruits are also great sources of fiber. So if you become constipated, it may simply be that you need to eat more vegetables and fruits as tolerated. In addition, adequate intake of natural fats, discussed later in this book, can also be helpful.

Occasionally, some people get very tired during or after the Two-Week Test. This can be due to a number of problems. Most commonly it's from not eating enough food, and/or not eating often enough. The most common problem is not eating breakfast. And many people should not go more than three to four hours without eating something healthy.

Case History

Bob was determined to renew his health in a natural way. He was overweight and overfat, always exhausted, and his blood pressure, cholesterol and triglycerides were too high. He started the Two-Week Test and initially felt very good. But within a few days he began getting tired and irritable. After talking with Bob for just a few minutes, it was clear that he was doing several things wrong. Because it caused him to spend more time in bathrooms, he did not drink much water during the day. In addition, since he thought about how many calories he was eating he became calorie conscious and ate less. To make matters worse, he thought that yogurt was in the cheese group, and was eating two or three containers of fruit yogurt each day. When I told Bob that the yogurt had 6 to 7 teaspoons of sugar in each container, and to forget about the calories for now and plan his water intake better, he started his test again. After the first week he was feeling great. Within a month, his energy remained high, and a couple of months after that, his visit to the doctor showed his blood pressure and blood fats were back to normal, and he had lost 14 pounds.

Maintaining Your Balance

Once you successfully finish the Two-Week Test, and add back the right amount of tolerable carbohydrate foods, you should have a very good idea of your carbohydrate limits — the amount of carbohydrate you can eat without producing symptoms. This is best accomplished by asking yourself about your signs and symptoms on a regular basis: energy, sleepiness and bloating after meals, etc. You may want to keep a diary so you can be more objective in your self-assessment. In time, you won't need to focus as much on this issue as your intuition will take over and you'll automatically know your limits.

Once you find your level of carbohydrate tolerance, you're on your way to balancing your whole diet. Now that you know how much carbohydrate you can tolerate, in the next chapter I'll discuss which types of carbohydrate foods are the healthiest to eat.

In review, here are the basics of the Two Week Test:

✔ Write a list of all your signs and symptoms.

✔ Weigh yourself.

✔ Plan your meals and snacks — buy sufficient foods allowed on the test, and get rid of those not allowed so you're not tempted.

✔ Eat as much as you need, and as often as you need to never get hungry.

✔ Always eat breakfast.

✔ After the test, re-evaluate your signs and symptoms, including weight.

✔ Begin adding natural, unprocessed carbohydrates to every other meal or snack, and evaluate whether this causes any of your previous signs or symptoms (including weight) to return.

✔ Enjoy your newfound health!

8

Carbohydrates: The Good and the Bad

After you determine the amount and type of healthy carbohydrates you can tolerate it's likely that these types of foods will remain a part of your diet. When choosing carbohydrate foods it's important to realize that not all are created equal. Some carbohydrates are more natural than others, thus the response they evoke in the body is less dramatic. In general, the more highly processed the carbohydrate food, the worse it is for you. Highly processed carbohydrates generally have a higher glycemic index than those that are processed less or not processed at all. Most commercially processed bread, bagels, rolls, cereals and other grain products, and those containing sugar, are so highly processed with virtually no nutritional value they can only harm your body and brain, impairing human performance. This does not mean you can't enjoy eating — in fact, there are many ways to create gourmet meals, including desserts, which are not only delicious but healthy.

So what carbohydrates should you eat? At the top of the list of unprocessed carbohydrates is fruit. In addition to containing vitamins and minerals, fruit also contains important phytonutrients. Though fruit is a carbohydrate food, the glycemic index of most fruit is low to moderate because fruit contains substantial amounts of fiber, and because fruit sugar, or fructose, has the lowest glycemic index of all sugars. Most fruits contain a combination of fructose and glucose, and those with the most fructose have a lower glycemic index. At the low end of the glycemic index are cherries, plums, grapefruits, apricots, cantaloupe, berries and peaches. Apples, pears and baby bananas have a more moderate glycemic index, with grapes, oranges and large bananas scoring higher. Pineapple, watermelon and dried fruits are among the highest-glycemic fruits and should be eaten sparingly, if at all. Most people who are CI can tolerate some amount of fresh fruits, although sometimes they can only eat from the low glycemic group.

Legumes or beans can be tolerated by many people, but often in small amounts. These foods are thought by many to be a protein food, but most contain much more carbohydrate than protein. For instance a serving of red beans typically may have 6 grams of protein and 16 grams of carbohydrate, with 5 of these carbohydrate grams as fiber. Because of the presence of both protein and fiber, the glycemic index of red beans and other legumes remains relatively low for a carbohydrate food. In addition, other legumes may have even lower glycemic effects. Overall, because of their composition, most beans, including lentils, have a moderate glycemic effect, and are a good alternative to refined-carbohydrate foods.

Vegetables also contain carbohydrates, though most have only small amounts. Vegetables are an extremely important item in the diet and are discussed in detail in a later chapter. Some vegetables, however, contain moderate to high amounts of carbohydrates and therefore warrant discussion here. Among the higher-carbohydrate vegetables are corn and potatoes, which should be eaten sparingly, if at all. In fact, a baked potato has a whopping 37 grams of carbohydrate — as much as a serving of cooked pasta — and a higher glycemic index than some cakes and candy. New potatoes have a much lower glycemic index than other varieties. The reason potatoes and corn are such high glycemic foods is because they have been genetically changed to be sweeter than the same foods a generation or two ago.

Many people consume the bulk of their carbohydrates as grains. Whole grains, and products made from them, are more healthful than their refined counterparts, and contain more of the nutrients and fiber from the original grain. For instance, whole oat groats are better than the common processed oatmeal cereals, especially the "quick" oats. Long-grain brown rice is better than short-grain white rice. Wild rice, which isn't really a rice but a seed from a reedy grass, is fairly low in carbohydrate and has a moderate glycemic index as well. There are a number of breads on the market made from whole, sprouted grains, and most have a lower glycemic index. Processed wheat flour (white flour) can increase insulin levels two to three times more than true whole-grain products. But whether whole or processed, grains are starches and more difficult to digest than most foods, and many people, often unknowingly, are intolerant to wheat of any kind. Wheat is such a common problem for many people that I devoted the section below to it.

Wheat: The Shaft of Life

Wheat may be the most unhealthy food staple of the Western diet next to sugar, contributing significantly to ill health and disease. We all know how bad sugar is for health due to its high glycemic nature — but wheat and wheat products can actually be worse due to an even higher glycemic index, so eating that piece of bread is not unlike eating a couple of spoons of white table sugar! And, much of this wheat, and sugar, turns to fat. For example, almost half of that so-called fat-free bagel can turn to stored fat.

Wheat is a lobbying success story, like the tobacco industry, as it's found in most people's media-driven diets. It's certainly not recommended for its nutritional reasons as we can obtain whatever benefits wheat contains (some fiber and nutrients) in many other healthy foods. And, considering the health risks, wheat's place on any food pyramid is a scheme that serves those who are addicted and the companies that sell it.

The facts are clear: Wheat is unhealthy. It's a common cause of intestinal problems, allergy and asthma, skin problems; it prevents absorption of various nutrients, contributes to weight gain and the obesity epidemic — and occasionally causes death.

The reason for wheat's failure as a healthy item is twofold; the protein component of wheat, called gluten, is highly allergenic in many people, including infants who are unfortunately given this as their first food. And many people are adversely affected by gluten without realizing it, with a slow, silent buildup of chronic illness. Gluten is what makes bread rise, so most baked goods and packaged foods are full of it.

The second reason wheat is unhealthy is that almost all wheat products are high glycemic — from bread, bagels and muffins to cereals and additives to many packaged foods to wheat flour itself, a staple in almost all kitchens and recipes. High-glycemic foods contribute to chronic disease, weight gain and other ills, and along with sugar wheat ranks among the worst.

Gone are the days when people would buy real whole-wheat berries, grind them and make flour or sprout them for use in food products. While the berries still contain gluten, they're not high glycemic. But almost all wheat used today is processed, making it high glycemic.

Consider too that wheat makes up a significant part of most people's diet. In doing so it also replaces many potentially healthy foods such as vegetables, fruits, protein foods such as eggs and meat, nuts and seeds, and others. For example, instead of unhealthy cereal for breakfast, a vegetable omelet would be a much healthier choice for most people.

The list of specific conditions associated with wheat keeps growing — from autoimmune diseases (such as arthritis, Type 1 diabetes, lupus, MS) and chronic inflammation to infertility and skin disorder (such as eczema, acne and psoriasis); and even cancer.

Some people are more sensitive to the harmful effects of wheat than others. Wheat allergy is among the common allergies in children and adults, along with milk, soy, peanuts and corn. The most practical way to assess this is to note how you feel after ingesting wheat. The most common symptom is intestinal bloating, but signs and symptoms are associated with skin, breathing and edema, and may be immediate or delayed. If you're sensitive to wheat, significantly reducing or eliminating it from your diet is the most effective remedy.

Here are some other points about how wheat can harm us:

- In the intestines, wheat can bind important minerals from food and prevent their absorption. These include calcium, magnesium, iron, zinc and copper — all essential for good health.

- Wheat can reduce digestive enzymes, especially those from the pancreas, rendering key foods less digestible — including protein and fats. By not digesting protein, amino acid absorption is impaired, and whole protein absorption could cause allergies. And by not digesting fat, essential fatty acids may not be absorbed, adversely affecting a whole spectrum of problems from skin quality to inflammation and hormonal balance.

- Since wheat is high glycemic, it can lead to the production of higher amounts of insulin by the pancreas. In addition to causing more fat storage, this can also increase your risk of various diseases including diabetes, cancer and heart disease.

- Combining exercise and wheat can trigger allergic reactions in some people, although it's not common. This occurs when a person eats some form of wheat, and exercises within a given time period. This is followed by some allergic reaction, from mild problems (sometimes so mild people are used to it) like skin rash or hives to more severe problems including anaphylaxis and even death. This may also include breathing difficulty. It is sometimes difficult to diagnose because of the need for both triggers (wheat and exercise) around the same time period. It's conceivable that some of the deaths reported in athletes are due to this problem.

- High-glycemic wheat products, which are often sweetened with more sugar, can result in a sweet-tooth — or addiction — that not only perpetuates the desire for more sweets, but the dislike for health-promoting less sweet-tasting and bitter foods, like vegetables.

- Wheat can sometimes cause mental or emotional symptoms, including depression, mood swings, attention problems in children and anxiety. Long-term illness associated with wheat allergy includes dementia due to cerebral (brain) atrophy.

- Osteoporosis may be strongly associated with wheat allergy.

- Other health issues can also be associated with wheat consumption. These include belching or gas, diarrhea or other abdominal discomfort; reduced mental focus and poor concentration, and fatigue — some people actually fall asleep after a meal containing wheat, even just a sandwich.

The extreme condition of wheat intolerance is celiac disease, and patients must avoid any amount of wheat or risk serious, sometimes life-threatening reactions. Many professionals now agree that even mild forms of wheat allergy are really the same thing — a sub-clinical celiac condition.

If you're in doubt about what wheat may be doing to your health, consider strictly avoiding it for a couple of weeks or a month. You just may become a new, healthier person.

What about Sweeteners?

Sweeteners are carbohydrates, or sugars, in their purest form. They range from highly processed and higher-glycemic products such as maltodextrin and table sugar, to the lower glycemic sources such as honey and agave nectar. As with other carbohydrate foods, the least processed and more natural sugars are the healthiest sweeteners.

Most sweeteners are complex carbohydrates — high glycemic and more difficult to digest. These include all maltose sugars (maltodextrin, malt sugar, maple sugar and syrup), corn sugars and syrups (high-fructose corn syrup), all cane sugars whether white or brown, rice syrups and molasses.

Perhaps the best sweeteners to use are low-glycemic simple carbohydrates that don't require digestion and are unprocessed. These include agave nectar and honey. I recommend honey for many reasons as discussed below, but in moderation and not to exceed your carbohydrate tolerance.

Honey has been used for centuries as both a sweetener and a remedy, and remains today as the most natural sweetener available. Honey contains a variety of vitamins, minerals and amino acids, including antioxidants. In addition, honey has anti-inflammatory and antimicrobial effects. Recently a large volume of scientific literature has substantiated honey's therapeutic value, as well as its ability to improve endurance in athletes.

Honey is also perhaps the only carbohydrate food that does not promote tooth decay through acidity. In general, proteins and fats raise salivary pH, making it more alkaline, while carbohydrate foods lower pH, making it more acidic. Honey is the sweet exception — a carbohydrate that may raise pH levels. In addition, honey has an overall beneficial effect on oral health due to its antibacterial effect and ability to reduce dextran, a sticky, sugary substance that helps bacteria adhere to the teeth.

Like fruit, honey is primarily a blend of fructose and glucose. Different types of honey have different ratios of each type of sugar. Those that crystallize fastest have the highest glucose content, and thus the higher glycemic index. Since fructose has the lowest glycemic index of all sugars, honey with higher fructose content will have the lowest glycemic index. Sage and tupelo honey, for example, are known for their high fructose content, while clover honey has a medium fructose content, and alfalfa honey is higher in glucose.

When shopping for honey, look for a number of attributes. Dark honey may be the most therapeutic and have the most nutrients. Buckwheat honey is said to contain the highest amounts of antioxidants. Raw, unfiltered honey retains more beneficial qualities. Heat, light and filtering remove some of the beneficial properties of honey.

Agave nectar is very high in fructose with a very low glycemic index. But it lacks the therapeutic benefits that honey contains. Due to its high fructose content, some individuals don't tolerate it. Intestinal distress is the most common symptom, and in those with high triglyceride levels, high fructose intake may worsen the condition.

What about Artificial Sweeteners?

I recommend avoiding artificial sweeteners in virtually all situations because I believe fake sugars can have an adverse effect on your health. Some say the research is still not clear on this issue. But I say why wait when there's enough information about it? Artificial sweeteners are used in many food items: diet soda, chewing gum, ice cream, iced-tea mixes and many other products. If you want to avoid them you must read the labels.

While substances such as saccharin are not recommended for children or pregnant women, and aspartame has been related to an increased incidence of migraine headaches and allergic reactions, another fact has been ignored: The use of artificial sweeteners is most often accompanied by increased consumption of food. In other words, if you use artificial sweeteners, studies show you often end up eating more food, usually sweets. What's worse is that you may store more fat as well. Researchers are unclear why this happens, but certain factors seem to be implicated. It may be a learned process by the body. The tasting of sweet substances may cause the body to store, rather than burn, fat. Or, it may be related to the dehydration that accompanies consumption of artificial sweeteners. This may trigger the brain to increase the appetite and food intake as a means of restoring water balance. Eating low-calorie substances will lower the body's metabolism. This will not only cause the body to store more fat but also activate the need to eat more food.

Some people argue that artificial sweeteners reduce calories. You may be fooled into believing that you are buying a more-healthful, low-calorie food when you choose a product made with fake sugar. But you're avoiding only 15 calories per teaspoon when using an artificial sweetener. This is not a significant caloric factor. Not only that, counting calories, as discussed elsewhere, is unhealthy.

Clearly if you want to be healthy and continually improve human performance, you need to understand how carbohydrates can affect overall health, especially in relation to your particular needs. In general, refined carbohydrates are best eliminated. The best choices are fruits, legumes and whole grains if tolerated, with small amounts of honey as a sweetener. As you begin to choose your carbohydrate foods more wisely, you will notice that you feel better. This is part of becoming more intuitive about your diet and individual needs. In addition to making wise choices about carbohydrate foods, you need to do the same when it comes to eating fat, which is discussed in the following chapters.

9

The Big Fat Lie

For decades, fat has been seen as the "bad" component of the diet. Low- and no-fat has become synonymous with being healthy. These ideas, of course, are untrue. In fact, fat is one of the most beneficial substances in your diet, and is often the missing ingredient in developing and maintaining optimal health and human performance. But an ongoing, well-financed misinformation campaign against fat has misled the public to an epidemic of fat phobia. Just think of the billions of dollars spent each year on low-fat and fat-free foods and you'll understand why you might not have been told the whole truth about fat. In addition, this anti-fat campaign has contributed to actual deficiencies in fat that have contributed to various diseases. The bottom line on dietary fat: Too much or too little is dangerous. It's simply a question of balancing your intake.

First, let's define fat — a term that also includes oil. Fats are found in concentrated forms such as vegetable oils, butter, egg yolk, cheese and other naturally occurring foods, and in less concentrated forms that make up the content of almost all natural foods. And some foods contain very small fat components that are as essential as all other nutrients.

Virtually all natural fats are healthy. As noted above, eating a balance of fats is most important. In general, eating too much of one type of fat, such as too much saturated fat from dairy products or too much omega-6 fat from vegetable oil, is an example of a fat imbalance that can adversely affect health. In addition, eating "bad" fats — those that are artificial and highly processed, such as trans fat and overheated fats in fried foods, can cause serious health problems. Foods such as chips, French fries and fried chicken, to name just a few, are examples of those containing bad fat.

Dietary fats have been a staple for humans throughout evolution. Ironically many people are learning of the true importance of fats in the diet only since the low-fat trend of the last few decades. This is not news, really. Scientists have known of the importance of fat in the diet since the discoveries in 1929 by researchers who demonstrated the necessity of dietary fat. Before discussing these issues — which fats are best and how can they be balanced — let's highlight some of the many healthy functions of fat.

- **Disease Prevention and Treatment.** Certain dietary fats consumed in balanced proportions can actually help prevent many diseases. For instance, we now know that dietary fats are central to controlling inflammation, which is the first stage of most chronic diseases. And, selectively increasing certain dietary fats has been shown to reduce the growth or spreading of cancer and improving recovery in heart disease. Many brain problems, including cognitive dysfunction such as Alzheimer's disease, can also be treated with fats. A healthy brain is more than 60 percent fat.

- **Energy.** The aerobic system depends on fat as the fuel for the aerobic muscles, which power us through the day. Fat produces energy, and prevents excessive dependency upon sugar, especially blood sugar. Fat provides more than twice as much potential energy as carbohydrates do, 9 calories per gram as opposed to only 4 calories. Your body is capable of obtaining much of its energy from fat, up to 80 or 90 percent, if your fat-burning mechanism is working efficiently. The body even uses fat as a source of energy for heart-muscle function. These fats — called phospholipids — normally are contained in the heart muscle and generate energy to make it work more efficiently.

- **Hormones.** The hormonal system is responsible for controlling virtually all healthy functions of the body. But for this system to function properly, the body must produce proper amounts of the appropriate hormones. These are produced in various glands, and dependent on fat for production of hormones. The adrenal glands, the thymus, thyroid, kidneys and other glands use fats to help make hormones. Cholesterol is one of the fats used for the production of hormones such as progesterone and cortisone. The thymus gland regulates immunity and the body's defense systems. The thyroid regulates temperature, weight and other metabolic functions. The kidney's hormones help regulate blood pressure, circulation and filtering of blood. Some hormonal problems are associated with body fat content that's too low. For example, some women with very low body fat, from too much exercise or very poor diet habits, experience disruptions in their menstrual cycle. In older women, this may also affect menopausal symptoms

- **Eicosanoids.** Hormone-like substances called eicosanoids, discussed in the next chapter, are necessary for such normal cellular function as regulating inflammation, hydration, circulation and free-radical activity. Produced from dietary fats, eicosanoids are especially important for their role in controlling inflammation — the precursor of many chronic diseases including cancer, heart disease and Alzheimer's. Many people who have inflammatory conditions, such as arthritis, colitis, tendinitis — conditions with names ending in "itis" — probably have an eicosanoid imbalance. But in many more people, chronic inflammation goes on silently. Eicosanoids are also important for regulating blood pressure and hydration. An imbalance can trigger constipation or diarrhea. Eicosanoid imbalance may also be associated with menstrual cramps, blood clotting, tumor growth and other problems.

- **Insulation.** The body's ability to store fat permits humans to live in most climates, especially in areas of extreme heat or cold. In warmer areas of the world, stored fat provides protection from the heat. In colder lands, increased fat stored beneath the skin prevents too much heat from leaving the body. An example of fat's effectiveness as an insulator is in the Eskimo's ability to withstand great cold and survive in good health. Eskimos eat a high-fat diet, and despite this have a very low incidence of heart disease and other ailments. In warmer climates, fat prevents too much water from leaving the body, which can result in dehydration that causes dry, scaly skin. Some evaporation is normal, of course, but fats under the skin regulate evaporation and can prevent as much as 10 to 20 times more water from leaving the body.

- **Healthy Skin and Hair.** Fat has protective qualities that also give skin the soft, smooth and unwrinkled appearance that many people try to achieve through expensive skin conditioners. The healthy look of skin comes from the fat inside. The same is true for your hair. Fats, including cholesterol, also serve as an insulating barrier within the skin. Without this protection, water and water-soluble substances such as chemical pollutants would enter the body through the skin. With the proper balance and amounts of fats in your diet, your skin and hair develop a healthy appearance. If you've been looking for the ideal skin and hair product, you can have it by balancing the fats in your diet.

- **Pregnancy and Lactation.** The effective functioning of the hormonal system is important to both would-be parents. Once conception does take place, fats are important to the continued good health of the mother and child. The uterus must maintain the health of the newly conceived embryo by providing nutrition until the placenta can begin to function, usually a period of a week or more. If there is an adequate level of progesterone, which is produced from fats, there should be enough nutrients for the embryo to survive the first critical week. Without enough progesterone, the embryo could die. The placenta must also form and produce hormones that affect the developing fetus. The estrogens and progesterone are fat-dependent and are produced in increasing quantities as the pregnancy continues. Together they promote the growth of the uterus and the storage of nutrients for the fetus. The proper development of the fetus has obvious hormonal relationships, which are dependent upon fats. Following birth, breastfeeding helps protect the baby against allergies, asthma and intestinal problems through its high fat content, particularly cholesterol. The baby is highly dependent upon the fat in the milk for survival, especially during the first few days. During this time, the fatty colostrum from breast milk is of vital nutritional importance.

- **Digestion.** Bile from the gall bladder is triggered by fat in the diet, which helps aid in the digestion and absorption of important fats and fat-soluble vitamins. Most of the fats in the diet are digested in the small intestine — a process that involves breaking the fat into smaller particles. The pancreas, liver, gall bladder and large intestine are also involved in the digestive process. Any of these organs not working properly could have an adverse impact on fat metabolism in general, but the two most important organs are the liver, which makes bile, and the pancreas, which make the enzyme lipase. Without sufficient fat in the diet, the gall bladder will not secrete enough bile for proper digestion. Fat also helps regulate the rate of stomach emptying. Fats in a meal slow stomach emptying, allowing for better digestion of proteins. If you are always hungry it may be because your meal is too low in fat and your stomach is emptying too rapidly. Fats also slow the absorption of sugar from the small intestines, which keeps insulin from rising too high and too quickly — essentially, fat in the meal lowers its glycemic index. Additionally, fats protect the inner lining of the stomach and intestines from irritating substances in the diet, such as alcohol and spicy foods.

- **Support and Protection.** Stored fat offers physical support and protection to vital body parts, including the organs and glands. Fat acts as a natural, built-in shock absorber, cushioning the body and its various parts from the wear and tear of everyday life, and helps prevent organs from sinking due to the downward pull of gravity. Fats also may protect the body against the harmful effects of X-rays. This occurs through physical protection of the cell, and by controlling free-radical production, generated as a result of X-ray exposure. In addition to medical X-rays, we are constantly exposed to X-rays from the atmosphere. This cosmic radiation penetrates most objects, including airplanes. The average person gets more cosmic radiation exposure during an airline flight from New York to Los Angeles than from a lifetime of medical X-rays.

- **Vitamin and Mineral Regulation.** Most people know that vitamin D is produced by exposure of the skin to the sun. However, it is actually cholesterol in the skin that allows this reaction to occur. Sunlight chemically changes cholesterol in the skin through the process of irradiation to vitamin D-3. This newly formed vitamin D is then absorbed into the blood, allowing calcium and phosphorous to be properly absorbed from the intestinal tract. Without the vitamin D, calcium and phosphorous would not be well absorbed and deficiencies of both could occur. But without cholesterol, the entire process would not occur. Besides vitamin D, other vitamins, including A, E and K, rely on fat for proper absorption and utilization. These important vitamins are present primarily in fatty foods, and the body cannot make an adequate amount of these vitamins to ensure continued good health. In addition these vitamins require fat in the intestines in order to be absorbed. So a low-fat diet could be deficient in these vitamins to begin with and also could further restrict their absorption. Certain fats are important for transporting calcium into the bones and muscles. Without this action, calcium levels in bones and muscles can be reduced resulting in the risk for stress fractures, osteoporosis, muscle cramps and other problems. Unused calcium may be stored, sometimes in the kidneys increasing the risk of stones, or in the muscles, tendons or joint spaces as calcium deposits.

- **Taste.** My favorite function of fat is that it makes food delightfully palatable. Want to make a recipe tastier? Add some healthy fat. Low- and no-fat products are usually quite bland, and often manufacturers add sugar to improve taste. Fat also satisfies your physical hunger by increasing satiety (the signal given to the brain that the meal is satisfying and you can stop eating). With a low-fat meal, the brain just keeps sending the same message over and over: Eat more! Because you never really feel satisfied, the temptation to overeat is irresistible. In fact, there's a good chance you can actually gain weight on a low-fat diet by overeating to try and get that "I'm not hungry anymore" feeling.

Types of Body Fat

The human body possesses two distinct types of body fat, referred to as brown and white. Both forms of body fat are active, living parts of us, heavily influencing our metabolism, protecting our organs, glands and bones, and offering many other health benefits mostly from our stores of white fat. This body fat content ranges from five percent in some male athletes to more than 50 percent of total body weight in obese individuals. Brown fat makes up only about 1 percent of the total body fat in healthy adults, although it's much more abundant at birth in healthy babies.

Brown fat helps us burn white fat; this is an important aspect of overall health. (Even in athletes, it's an important energy source for better performance.) Without adequate brown fat, we can gain body fat and become sluggish in the winter like a hibernating animal. There are a number of ways to increase brown fat activity.

Certain foods can stimulate brown fat and increase overall fat-burning. Eating several times a day, five to six smaller healthy meals instead of one, two or three larger ones, for example, can trigger a process called thermogenesis — an important post-meal metabolic stimulation for fat-burning. However, if caloric intake is too low, brown fat can slow the burning of white fat. This can happen on a low-calorie diet and when we skip meals.

Brown fat is also stimulated by certain dietary fats. The best ones are omega-3 fats, especially from fish oil, and olive oil (use olive to replace all vegetable oils in the diet).

This works in part because a moderately high healthy-fat diet can stimulate brown fat.

Other foods that increase brown fat activity include caffeine. Tea, coffee and chocolate contain small to high amounts of caffeine. However, if under stress, the adrenal glands become overworked, which can promote fat storage and reduce fat-burning; caffeine may worsen adrenal stress in many individuals. Also, avoid coffee, tea and chocolate products if they contain sugar, which can reduce fat-burning.

While supplements of fish oil may be the only way to obtain adequate amounts of EPA, some supplements can be harmful. A popular supplement, CLA (conjugated linoleic acid), can actually reduce brown fat activity.

Brown fat is greatly controlled by skin temperature. If you get too hot during the day, or overdress during exercise, brown-fat activity can lead to less burning of white fat. This is why exercising in extra clothes or "sweatsuits," a common but unhealthy weight-loss routine, can be dangerous.

Even sitting in a hot tub, sauna or steam room regularly after exercise may offset some of the fat-burning benefits of physical activity. These activities can increase sweating, resulting in some water-weight loss, but the sacrifice is actually less fat-burning. Hot tubs and saunas do come with health benefits, but to avoid the reductions in fat-burning take a minute or two to cool the body in a cold shower or tub afterwards.

In contrast, brown fat is stimulated by cold. Cooling the body's brown-fat areas can help stimulate more fat-burning. Brown fat is found around the shoulders and underarms, between the ribs and at the nape of the neck. These are important areas to keep from over-heating and cool after exercise. (Low *body temperature* is associated with reduced fat-burning; this is often related to low thyroid function.)

Of course, exercise can increase fat-burning too. The best kind being the easy aerobic type, such as walking, which trains the body to burn more body fat all day and night. This issue is discussed in detail in later chapters.

Unfortunately, most research in the area of brown fat comes from the pharmaceutical industry, which is looking for a new drug to stimulate brown fat. But a healthy diet, the right exercise and other lifestyle habits already can do this!

The role of brown fat is just another of the many examples of healthy functions of fat in the body. But to make sure we have healthy, balanced fats, we must be very careful with the types and amounts of fats we consume.

It's time to look at fat as our friend. Good fats can greatly help in the quest to improve optimal health and human performance.

10

Balancing Your Fats

Now that we've discussed the importance of natural dietary fats for human performance and the necessity of healthy body fat, it's just as important to outline how to balance your consumption of certain fats in the diet. It's accomplished in three simple steps. When using fats and oils:

- For cooking, use only olive oil, butter, coconut oil or lard.

- Avoid all vegetable oil and trans fat.

- Balance consumption of omega-6 and omega-3 fats in a 2:1 ratio.

The issue of balancing fat consumption is quite complex; volumes have been written on the subject and many scientists have devoted their entire careers to this topic. But I have simplified the explanations to help you achieve this important task. First, let's look at three common types of fats: monounsaturated, polyunsaturated and saturated.

Monounsaturated Fat

This fat is associated with improved health and disease prevention and should make up the bulk of fat in your diet. Monounsaturated fat, also referred to as oleic or omega-9, has been shown to have many health benefits, including helping prevent cancer, heart disease, obesity and other chronic illnesses. The Mediterranean diet, with its lower incidence of obesity and diseases, is relatively high in monounsaturated fat, which may be the key reason for the health benefits. In some cases, we know how monounsaturated fat can prevent disease. For example, this fat is known to raise "good" HDL cholesterol and lower "bad" LDL cholesterol, which can greatly improve cardiovascular health.

Monounsaturated fat is also very stable. As discussed later, polyunsaturated fat is easily oxidized and can form dangerous oxygen free radicals from exposure to air, light and heat. These free radicals can lead to bodily dysfunction and even disease. Due to its chemical structure, monounsaturated fat is virtually immune to oxidation through cooking or exposure to air and light.

Monounsaturated fat is found in many foods, and some oils are predominantly this type of fat. Foods highest in monounsaturated fats are avocados, almonds and macadamia nuts, with other nuts and seeds containing moderate amounts. Olive oil is very high in monounsaturated fat and is the best oil for both cooking and use on salads or other foods.

The best olive oil to use is the least processed and most nutritious — extra virgin olive oil. This is obtained from the whole fruit by using the cold-press technique, which does not alter the natural antioxidants, phytonutrients or quality of the oil. The most potent phytonutrients are phenols, which give the oil its slight bitter taste. Very high amounts of phenols are found in extra-virgin olive oil. Phytonutrients, including phenols, are virtually absent in almost all other oils, including olive oils that are not extra-virgin. The benefits of phytonutrients are discussed in more detail in a later chapter.

Most olive oil comes from Spain, Greece and Italy. Graded by international standards, much like fine wine, for flavor, aroma and acidity, extra-virgin olive oil is the tastiest and has less than 1 percent natural acid. Highly acidic oils (above 3.3 percent acidity) have an offensive taste and are neutralized by added chemical agents, so avoid other forms of olive oil including "pure" and "light" versions.

By using extra-virgin olive oil for most of your oil needs, as well as eating foods that are high in health-promoting monounsaturated fat such as avocados and almonds, you'll be taking an important step to balancing your dietary fats.

Polyunsaturated Fat

Many foods naturally contain polyunsaturated fat. They include omega-6 and omega-3 essential fatty acids that play a vital role in regulating inflammation as well as performing other key functions. Concentrated and potentially dangerous amounts of omega-6 fat are in vegetable oil, with the highest levels contained in safflower, peanut, corn, canola and soy oil, and many processed foods including infant formulas. Too much omega-6 polyunsaturated fat, whether from vegetable oil, processed food or dietary supplements, can adversely affect health in two significant ways. First, an excess of omega-6 oil can convert to a fatty acid called arachidonic acid. Too much of this fatty acid may contribute significantly to chronic inflammation, the first stage of all chronic diseases and other problems. This is detailed below.

Second, polyunsaturated fat is easily oxidized to chemical free radicals, making it a potentially dangerous food. Oxidation occurs when this type of fat is heated, or exposed to light and air. When we consume oxidized fat, this free-radical stress can damage cells anywhere in the body, speed the aging process, turn LDL cholesterol "bad" and significantly increase the need for antioxidant nutrients. The fat content of most people's diet is very high in concentrated omega-6 fats from vegetable oils and dairy products, a serious imbalance.

One way to make polyunsaturated fat work toward optimal health, rather than contributing to disease, is to balance consumption. To accomplish better balance, avoid all vegetable oils and processed food; instead, use extra-virgin olive or other recommended fats. Before discussing this issue in more detail, let's discuss saturated fat because it's part of the balancing act.

Saturated Fat

Of all the dietary fats, saturated fat is always considered the least healthful. But saturated fat is important for energy and hormone production, cellular functioning and other important actions much like other fats.

Like other fat, saturated forms are made up of many different fatty acids, some of which have been linked to ill health when consumed in excess. The worst may be palmitic acid, high in dairy fat. This fatty acid can raise cholesterol, and some of the dietary carbohydrate that converts to fat becomes palmitic acid. High blood levels of palmitic acid may predict type 2 diabetes, heart disease, stroke and carbohydrate intolerance. However, when fats are balanced, palmitic acid does not seem to be such a health problem. (Palm-kernel oil is also high in palmitic acid, but palm-fruit oil is not, and actually contains important tocotrienols that can lower LDL cholesterol.)

Arachidonic acid — AA — is another component of saturated fat that gives it a bad name. While small amounts are essential for health, high AA levels are very unhealthy. AA is found in dairy, egg yolks, meats and shellfish. However, the amounts in these foods are relatively small compared to the amount of AA produced by the conversion of omega-6 fatty acids from vegetable oils in the average diet. Like many other situations regarding fat, balance is the key. In the case of AA, it's an essential fatty acid, especially for the brain, for the fetus, newborns and growing children. But in larger amounts it can cause problems. Too much AA, either from saturated fat or vegetable oil, can create chronic inflammation, bone loss, increased pain and other problems discussed later.

The good side of saturated fat is important too. Stearic acid, for example, has various health benefits for the immune system. This saturated fatty acid is found in cocoa butter and grass-fed beef. And, stearic acid can be converted within the body to monounsaturated fat. Another healthy saturated fatty acid is lauric, which plays an important role in energy production and has anti-viral and anti-bacterial actions, especially in the intestine (and the stomach in particular, against H. pylori). Coconut oil, high in saturated fat, is also high in healthy lauric acid (and contains very little polyunsaturated fat, making it an ideal fat for cooking).

In animal foods, which contain relatively high amounts of saturated fat, the most important factor that determines the fatty acid profile is the food consumed by the animal. Grass-fed beef, for example, contains a much healthier content of fatty acids compared to corn-fed beef. For the same reason, wild animals usually contain healthier fatty-acid profiles than animals that are fed grain in confinement. In plants, the soil plays a certain role in determining fatty acid content.

Before discussing a key feature in balancing dietary fats, it's worth looking at the fat content of various foods to demonstrate the mixture of mono, poly and saturated fat in each. A few foods contain predominantly one type of fat or another, but most foods, even oils, contain a combination of all three. Many people are surprised to learn, for instance, that the fat in an average steak is about half monounsaturated and half saturated, with a small amount of polyunsaturated.

The following table shows approximately how much of each type of fat is contained in some foods.

Food	% Mono	% Poly	% Saturated
Olive oil	77	9	14
Canola oil	62	32	6
Peanut oil	49	33	18
Corn oil	25	62	13
Soybean oil	24	61	15
Safflower oil	13	77	10
Coconut	6	2	92
Egg yolks	48	16	36
Steak	49	4	47
Cheese	30	3	67
Butter	30	4	66
Almonds	68	22	10
Cashews	61	18	21
Peanuts	50	32	18

The ABCs of Fats: Optimal Balance

Together, polyunsaturated and saturated fats contain three important fatty acids I'll call A, B and C fats. In the body, each of these fats is converted to .three different groups of hormone-like substances called eicosanoids (pronounced i-cos-an-oids). I'll call these groups 1, 2 and 3. Basically, A fats make group 1 eisosanoids, B fats group 2, and C fats group 3. This is a very simplified explanation, but fairly accurate; and it's important to understand the basics of fat metabolism because of its powerful effect on overall health and human performance. All these fats are important for optimal health. But when there's an imbalance, the result is reduced health and higher risk of disease.

An imbalance of eicosanoids resulting in too much of group 2 promotes inflammation, pain, bone loss, muscle problems, allergy, asthma, and potentially, disease such as cancer, Alzheimer's, diabetes,

The ABCs of Fats		
A Fats	**B Fats**	**C Fats**
↓	↓	↓
Group 1 Eicosanoids	**Group 2 Eicosanoids**	**Group 3 Eicosanoids**

stroke and heart disease. The right balance of eicosanoids can prevent, postpone, and even treat these conditions. Eicosanoid balance is so powerful — so influential to overall health — that billions of dollars are spent by pharmaceutical companies to research and develop new drugs that attempt to balance the eicosanoids. But you can do it for pennies by eating the right foods! And while drugs that attempt to balance fats have some short-term success, they come with significant unhealthy, and sometimes deadly, side effects. Balancing fats by eating right only has healthy — nearly miraculous — benefits.

The term eicosanoid is a general one that encompasses a variety of very different compounds with names such as prostaglandins, leukotrienes and thromboxanes. They're involved in complex reactions from moment to moment in all cells throughout the body. For now just remember that balanced eicosanoids regulate certain bodily functions that are central to optimal human performance and disease prevention. With this in mind, understanding how to balance the A, B and C fats, and the 1, 2 and 3 groups of eicosanoids, is vital. First let's discuss A, B and C fats in more detail.

A fats are found in vegetables with the highest amounts in their oils: safflower, soy, corn, peanut and canola. These fats are referred to as omega-6, and contain an essential fatty acid called linoleic acid that I'll call LA for short. Like all essential fatty acids, they are "essential" because the body can't make them and we must eat them to be healthy. When we do, LA is converted to other fats, including GLA (gamma-linolenic acid), with the end result being the series 1 eicosanoids. These are powerful substances for promoting and maintaining health. Among the benefits are powerful anti-inflammation effects that can reduce the risk of many problems and prevent chronic illness throughout the body. Common dietary supplements of omega-6 products include black-currant-seed, borage and primrose oils that contain high amounts of GLA.

While group 1 eicosanoids from A fats can produce powerful health effects, there are potential problems. One is that conversion of A fats to group 1 can be impaired by a variety of things; these include reduced nutrients, including niacin, vitamin B6, magnesium, protein and others. In addition, trans fats can reduce the conversion, as can too much stress. And, as we age, the process tends to slow down. The remedy? Eat the best diet possible to ensure you obtain all the nutrients, avoid bad fats and moderate stress (a topic discussed in detail in later chapters).

Another more serious problem is that, as noted above, A fats can convert to B fats and inflammatory eicosanoids, which can wreck health and destroy human performance if produced in excess. These are the B fats and group 2 eicosanoids.

The B fats are sometimes considered bad fats because of the effects they can have in the body. But these effects are only bad when in excess. B fats contain the essential fat AA (arachidonic acid), as noted above, and produce group 2 eicosanoids. Among the effects these eicosanoids promote are inflammation and pain. But these so-called problems can actually be important for health at the right time. For example, inflammation is a vital first stage of the healing process. Following this acute inflammatory process, as healing proceeds, anti-inflammatory eisocanoids in group 1 and 3 are produced to reduce inflammation. Another example is pain; the body uses pain to help you be aware of problems so you can remedy it. Chronic pain is not normal, or healthy, and usually associated with an unresolved problem associated with an imbalance of eicosanoids.

Another important function of AA (which is also considered an omega-6 fat) is that it's very important for the repair and growth of the brain. This is especially vital in the fetus, newborns and developing children, but as adults, we continually should be repairing and growing the brain as well.

B fats are highest in dairy products such as butter, cream and cheese, and in lesser amounts in the fat of meats, egg yolks and shellfish. However, for most people, the largest source of AA is from A fats. This is especially a problem when too many A fats are consumed, usually from vegetable oils, or if too much GLA is taken as a supplement. By eliminating vegetable oil and using only olive or coconut oil, the overall balance of fats is usually greatly improved. In addition to the common use at home, vegetable oils are often used in packaged foods and in restaurants.

The C fats are termed omega-3, and are found mostly in ocean fish, with lesser amounts in beans, flaxseed and walnuts. Smaller amounts are found in vegetables and wild and grass-fed animals. These fats contain ALA (alpha-linolenic acid), an essential fatty acid that is converted in the body to EPA (eicosapentaenoic acid), with the final production of group 3 eicosanoids. This conversion can be impaired by the same problems that impair the conversion of A fats to group 1 eicosanoids — poor nutrition, trans fat, stress and aging.

Fish oils derived from cold-water ocean fish already contain EPA and are very useful for people who require an omega-3 supplement to balance fats. Flaxseed oil is also common, but does not contain EPA and therefore requires other nutritional factors to convert to EPA. And, in humans, conversion of flax to EPA is very inefficient. Flax oil is also very unstable and can turn unhealthy if not fresh and refrigerated. (EPA also exists in conjunction with another important fatty acid, DHA, which is especially important for the fetus through childhood.)

It's relatively easy to balance A, B and C fats to promote a balance of the 1, 2 and 3 groups of eicosanoids. This can be accomplished first by eating approximately equal amounts of A, B and C fats. It does not necessarily have to be at each meal, but in the course of a day or week, balance is of prime importance. And, by eating a balance of A, B and C fats, you'll consume polyunsaturated and saturated fats in the optimal ratio of 2:1. In the typical Western diet, many people consume ratios of 5, 10 or even 20:1! It's no wonder there's an epidemic of pain and chronic disease. (If you don't eat meat or dairy, consume approx-

The ABCs of Fat: A Summary			
Type of Fat	A	B	C
Food source:	vegetable oils	animal fats	fish, flax
Contains:	LA	AA	ALA
Converts to:	GLA		EPA
Eicosanoids:	Group 1	Group 2	Group 3

imately an equal ratio of A and C fats; in this case, some of the A fats will convert to B fats.)

Fat imbalance typically occurs from some combination of eating too much A or B fats, and too little C fats; but it can also can be affected by certain foods, vitamins and drugs. The most common food that does this is refined carbohydrates, including sugar. Recall that insulin can be produced in higher amounts when these carbohydrates are consumed. This causes more A fats to convert to B fats, as AA, and into the group 2 eicosanoids. This is another reason refined carbohydrates are so unhealthy. Two foods can prevent too much A fats from converting to group 2 eicosanoids. These are EPA found in fish, and raw sesame oil, which contains the phytonutrient sesamin.

An important item mentioned above is that a number of other dietary and lifestyle factors can impair the conversion of A and C fats to their respective group 1 and 3 eicosanoids as summarized in the following table:

Factors that <u>Increase</u> Group 1 & 3 Eicosanoids	Factors that <u>Inhibit</u> Group 1 & 3 Eicosanoids
Vitamins B6, C and niacin, low doses of vitamin E, magnesium, zinc and calcium, alcohol in moderation	Trans fats, excess B fats, stress, aging, high-glycemic carbohydrates, low-protein diet, cigarette smoke, fever

A Note about Inflammation

I've mentioned inflammation often in this book so far, and will continue to do so (including a whole separate chapter) because it's such an important issue. Balancing the body's inflammatory/anti-inflammatory mechanism can help you attain optimal health and human performance — that's what balancing fats is all about.

Inflammation is the body's way of responding to and repairing itself from daily wear and tear, and injury. For example, just going for a walk, working on the computer, washing the dishes, or any other repetitive motion, not to mention exercise, produces chemicals that cause inflammation as part of the body's complex recovery process. More serious injury produces inflammation, too — a cut hand, a damaged joint, or an irritated stomach. The reddish, swollen, hot area of a cut finger is an example of this normal inflammatory process. Once the initial inflammation (from group 2 eicosanoids) has got the healing under way, anti-inflammatory chemicals (groups 1 and 3) are produced to stop the inflammation process and allow the healing to be completed.

One problem with this mechanism is that sometimes the cause of the initial problem is never resolved. For example, continued physical overuse of the shoulder, or irritation of the stomach with too much alcohol, perpetuates inflammation because the body is not allowed to heal. Another common problem is that the body is unable to make sufficient anti-inflammatory substances because there is too little group 1 and 3 eicosanoids; or there is too much of the inflammatory group 2 eicosanoids.

When inflammation becomes chronic a variety of end result signs and symptoms prevail, from arthritis and colitis to chronic muscle and joint injuries. Along the way, the process of disease may also develop. In time, the end result may be any type of ulcer or cancer, heart disease, cognitive brain disorders such as Alzheimer's and other chronic illness. Quality of life is greatly diminished and health and human performance are gradually destroyed.

Anti-inflammatory Drugs

In the conversion of A, B and C fats to eicosanoids, an important enzyme called cyclooxygenase, or COX, is required. There are actually two COX enzymes, and many people are familiar with the term "COX-2 inhibitors." These are drugs that act on these enzymes. Aspirin, and all other non-steroidal anti-inflammatory drugs (NSAIDS), including Advil, Motrin, Naprosyn and Nuprin, temporarily block the COX enzyme, so much less of the inflammatory series 2 eicosanoids are formed. While this reduces the inflammatory group 2 eicosanoids, these drugs can also eliminate groups 1 and 3, along with their beneficial properties. This may result in an improvement of symptoms, but it also turns off the important anti-inflammatory mechanism. In addition, the cause of the problem — fat imbalance — goes untreated. If aspirin makes you feel better, it usually indicates that your fats are not balanced.

In addition to controlling inflammation and pain, eicosanoids have many other important functions. Both groups 1 and 3 decrease blood clotting and dilate blood vessels, which lowers blood pressure and increases circulation. Group 2 eicosanoids, however, do almost the opposite, increasing blood clotting, constricting blood vessels and increasing blood pressure. But these activities can be healthy when balanced. For example, without the constricting of blood vessels and the raising of blood pressure during stress, blood circulation would be poor and not enough oxygen and other nutrients would be circulated to where these things are needed. Or, without blood clotting, you could bleed to death from a small cut. Balance is key.

But excess group 2 eicosanoids can be deadly: they constrict blood vessels too much, and clot blood too much. They can also trigger tumor growth, atherosclerosis (fat deposits), asthma and allergy, bone loss and even promote menstrual cramps.

Many people are unaware that their fats are not balanced. Certain signs, symptoms and lifestyle habits may offer powerful clues that your eicosanoids may be out of balance. The following survey can help you determine the likelihood that you have an imbalance in fats and eicosanoids. Check the items below that apply to you:

❏ Aspirin or non-steroidal anti-inflammatory drugs improve symptoms.

❏ Chronic inflammation or "itis"-type conditions such as arthritis, colitis, tendinitis.

❏ History or increased risk of heart disease, stroke or high blood pressure.

❏ Often eat restaurant, take-out or fast food.

❏ Low-fat diet.

❏ Feelings of depression.

❏ History of tumors or cancers.

❏ Periods of reduced mental acuity.

❏ Diabetes or family history of diabetes.

❏ Over age 50.

❏ Blood tests show increased triglycerides or cholesterol.

❏ Carbohydrate intolerance.

❏ Seasonal allergies.

❏ Intestinal problems such as diarrhea, constipation, ulcers.

If you checked one or more of these items there's a chance that you have a fat imbalance. The more items you check off, the more likely you have a problem.

Most people find they are too high in A and B fat and low in C fats because omega-6 fat and dairy foods are so prevalent in most diets. This can be remedied by balancing dietary fats — eating less A and more C fats. The greatest problem for many people is consuming enough C fats, especially EPA. Most foods high in C fats such as almonds, walnuts, pecans, flaxseeds and green vegetables, don't contain EPA and their conversion to EPA is very limited in humans, so we must rely on fish. Wild ocean fish — including salmon, sardines, tuna, anchovies and mackerel — are high in EPA. Unfortunately, the world's oceans continue to be seriously polluted, especially with mercury, and fish intake should be limited, especially by children and pregnant women. Farmed fish should be avoided — they are a poor source of EPA and have other problems discussed in a later chapter.

One remedy that can significantly help balance fats is fish-oil supplements. These contain high amounts of EPA, and in combination with reducing vegetable oils can make fat balance a reality. EPA also helps prevent some of the A fats from converting to B fats. In addition, raw sesame-seed oil helps prevent this process too. Be sure to buy small amounts of only raw sesame oil, don't cook it, and keep it refrigerated because it's a relatively unstable polyunsaturated oil.

How Much Fat Should We Eat?

Equipped with the knowledge of how important balanced fats are for the body, you are in a position to improve your diet in accordance with your body's particular needs. How much fat should you have in a healthy diet? The amount of fat in a healthy diet depends on the individual.

You must first get over the idea that the less fat the better, or a diet that's 10 percent or 20 percent fat is ideal. Actually, a low-fat diet can be very unhealthy. For example, studies show that people following a very low-fat diet can increase their risks for heart disease. This is due to the fact that their intake of essential fatty acids could be too low. There are many populations in which fat intake exceeds 40 percent, like the Eskimos and people living in the Mediterranean region, who on average are healthier than people who eat a lower-fat diet. In addition, the American Heart Association, the World Health Organization (WHO), the Surgeon General, the USDA and many professional health organizations have recommended a diet that's 30 percent fat.

I have found that most people are healthier with at least this much fat in the diet. Some may need more — 35 or even 40 percent. But rather than follow these numbers, experiment and find what works best for you. In general, once you've found your optimal level of carbohydrates, and balanced your fats, the amount of protein you need to eat is fairly easy to determine; this is the subject of the next chapter.

11

The Power of Protein

Once you've determined the right amount of carbohydrates for your body, and balanced your fats, proper protein intake is relatively easy to determine. For example, if you find that 40 percent of your macronutrients are carbohydrates, and 30 percent fat, the remaining 30 percent as protein would probably be the optimal amount for you. As convenient and oversimplified as that may sound, that's how it turns out for most people. Find the first two pieces of the puzzle and the third falls neatly into place.

However, there's no need to determine percentages — or grams, calories or any other quantity. Instead, make the appropriate changes as outlined in these chapters, beginning with carbohydrates, and let it all fall into place; your intuition will become a powerful ally. Coralee Thompson, M.D., simplifies protein needs even more. "At each meal eat the amount of dense protein food such as meat, fish or eggs that fits in the palm of your hand."

We all need protein every day for optimal health and increased human performance. This is true at all ages, for males and females, and whether you are walking 30 minutes a day or training for a 1,000-mile race.

Larger body frames and those performing a lot of physical work usually need more protein. Growing children also need relatively higher amounts of protein for development. In fact, throughout life there is still a significant and continuous need for protein.

Protein is necessary for so many healthy bodily functions, discussing it all would fill several books. Here are just a few examples:

- Enzymes important for balancing fats, digestion and hundreds of other metabolic activities necessary for optimal health require protein.

- Protein is essential for maintaining neurotransmitters — the chemical messengers used by the brain, the rest of the nervous system and gut for communication.

- Protein is a key element for building new cells, especially for muscles, bones, organs and glands, throughout life.

- Oxygen, fats, vitamins, hormones and other compounds are regulated and transported throughout the body with the help of protein.

- Protein is necessary to make natural antibodies for the immune system.

- Protein contains key amino acids for health. For example, cysteine is necessary for the body to make its most powerful antioxidant, glutathione, and glutamine is used to fuel the intestine for optimal function, especially for digestion and absorption of nutrients.

- Protein is important for the production of glucagon in relation to controlling insulin and blood sugar.

Studies continue to show that the protein recommendations by the USDA are too low. These recommendations have resulted in reductions in protein intake by some people, with dire health consequences. Even the argument that protein can harm the kidneys, especially those with kidney problems, is losing ground as new studies show that restricting dietary protein in those with kidney problems can actually increase the risk of death.

Most of this confusion about protein requirements comes from old and outdated research. When determining protein needs, researchers measured the amount of protein taken in through food, then measured protein by-products to determine the amount lost. Many studies on protein requirements, especially research that established today's RDA levels, only measured the protein by-product nitrogen, excreted in the urine. They failed to consider the amount lost in sweat. This is clearly an important means for excreting the nitrogen from protein breakdown. Urea production alone may not accurately reflect all aspects of protein breakdown. This is one reason many earlier studies on protein requirements showed such low numbers. Today, there are better, more accurate ways of determining protein needs through more elaborate measurements. These show that for most people, protein needs are higher than the old recommendations indicate.

How Much Protein?

The answer to this question depends on you — your lean body mass, your level of physical activity and other factors, including what makes you feel best. There is a wide range of healthy and safe protein intake that can provide many benefits. In addition to what has already been stated about finding your protein needs, for those who still need help understanding this important issue I'll discuss protein needs in grams using the USDA's recommendations to further put this subject into perspective.

The problem with this level of protein is that it's the bare minimum for an inactive person. And, it's based on body weight and not lean muscle mass. This amount is 0.8 grams of dietary protein per kilogram (2.2 pounds) of body weight. Based on this, a person weighing about 70 kilograms or 150 pounds should consume 60 grams of protein per day. This can be obtained with two eggs at breakfast, a salad with fish at lunch and a small steak at dinner.

But for most active, healthy people, this amount is insufficient. Recent studies show that protein requirements should be twice that of the USDA suggestion. Based on these studies performed over the past several years, and my clinical experience, I prefer to recommend a range of normal that includes the minimum amount of 0.8 grams to about 1.6 grams per kilogram of body weight. For most athletes, and those with very physical jobs, the amount of protein may still need to be increased above this level. Those involved in jogging/running, biking, swimming and other aerobic-type exercise, usually need more protein because the normal continual process of building muscle may actually be greater than that of weight-lifters.

For most active, healthy people, a normal protein intake over 1.0 grams per kilogram of body weight, usually closer to the 1.6 number, is best. Following are some examples of food servings that provide these amounts of protein:

- For a 175-pound person, the daily protein intake may be 128 grams. The protein foods that would provide this include three eggs and cheese at breakfast, a salad with a hefty serving of turkey at lunch and salmon for dinner.

- For a 145-pound person, the requirement may be about 106 grams: two eggs for breakfast, a chef's salad for lunch and a sirloin steak for dinner.

- And for the person weighing 125 pounds, who would minimally require about 90 grams of protein: two eggs at breakfast, tuna salad for lunch and lamb for dinner.

If you're 200 pounds or more, or appreciably under 125 pounds, just estimate the protein requirements based on the above numbers. For example, at 200 pounds, that's 25 percent heavier, so 25 percent more than 128 grams of protein is 160 grams.

Clearly, eating more protein than the body can utilize can be unhealthy. But if you require more than 100 grams a day, that's not excessive, it's what your body needs. Eating the amount of protein your body requires is not a high-protein diet, it's getting your proper requirements!

Sometimes, when unhealthy people consume normal amounts of protein they won't feel good because something else is wrong. For example, as protein intake increases, so does your need for water, which helps eliminate the normal by-products of protein through the kidneys. That's part of the old argument that protein is a stress on the kidneys; it most certainly is if you are dehydrated.

Or, if you're under significant stress and your stomach does not make sufficient amounts of natural hydrochloric acid — the first chemical stage of protein digestion — protein digestion can be a problem that could give you symptoms of intestinal distress. Addressing the cause of the problem — the stress and stomach, not the protein — is the best remedy. Or, another potential protein problem may occur if you combine a steak with some bread or a potato — this is a significant stress for the stomach, and indigestion often follows.

Amino Acids

Just as carbohydrates are made up of sugars, and fats are composed of fatty acids, dietary protein is made up of building blocks called amino acids. In order to obtain these vital components, the intestine must do its job. First, protein must be efficiently digested in the intestine, resulting in breakdown into amino acids. Second, these amino acids must be absorbed into the body. Once absorbed, the amino acids are used either as individual products, or recombined as proteins. For example, the amino acid tryptophan is used to make certain neurotransmitters in the brain. Or, recombining many amino acids provides for the manufacture of new muscle cells.

There are at least 20 amino acids necessary to human nutrition, all of which are indispensable for optimal health and human performance. While some amino acids can be manufactured in the body by other raw materials from food, others called "essential amino acids" must be taken in through the diet. While amino acids that are made in the body are sometimes referred to as "non-essential," this is misleading as all amino acids are essential.

In general, animal foods are the best sources of protein and contain all the amino acids. Overall, the highest-rated protein food is eggs, followed by beef and fish. With the exception of soybeans, which are mostly carbohydrate, vegetable foods individually contain only some of the amino acids. Combining the right non-animal foods can provide a complete amino-acid meal. But eating all the amino acids at one meal is not necessary.

For those who don't eat animal products, obtaining all the amino acids is accomplished by combining enough variety, since no one plant-based food, except soybeans, contains all the amino acids (although soy is very low in the amino acid methionine). Certain combinations of plant foods, such as beans and rice, or whole grains and legumes, can provide a complete protein. However, combining meals high in carbohydrates (such as rice, beans, grains, etc.) with protein can reduce digestibility, with the result that some protein will not digest into amino acids, and some amino acids won't get absorbed. This is discussed in a later chapter. In the next chapter I'll discuss some of best ways to obtain protein from the diet.

12

Making Wise Protein Choices

For most people getting enough protein should not be a problem as there are many healthy options. These include eggs, meats, fish and dairy foods. For those who won't eat these foods, getting enough protein can be a challenge. Soybeans and certain combinations of legumes and grains can supply all essential amino acids, but you risk not getting adequate protein, and generally must eat more carbohydrate than needed. For most people obtaining sufficient protein is relatively easy, especially when choosing animal sources.

Choosing the best animal proteins means finding the best sources. This may be organic, grass-fed, free-range, kosher and whatever other labels are used to differentiate the highest quality eggs, meats, fish and dairy foods from those obtained from poorly treated animals. In some cases, visiting a smaller local farm, for example, will help you decide. Some of today's local farmers are not only health-conscious but actually care about their animals and how their operations impact the environment.

The human body, especially the intestine, is well adapted for digesting animal-source foods, having evolved on a high-meat/fish, low-carbohydrate diet with varying amounts of vegetables, fruits and nuts. While the popular trend in recent decades has been toward the misconception that meat consumption is unhealthy, there are a variety of unique features of an animal-food diet that are vital for health and fitness. Here are some of them:

- Animal foods contain high levels of all essential amino acids.

- Vitamin B12 is an essential nutrient found only in animal foods.

- EPA, the most powerful fatty acid, and the one preferred by the human body, is almost exclusively found in animal foods.

- Iron deficiency is a common worldwide problem and is prevented by eating animal foods, which contain this mineral in its most bioavailable form.

- Vitamin A is found only in animal products (conversion of beta carotene in plant foods to vitamin A is not always efficient in humans).

- Animal products are dense protein foods with little or no carbohydrate to interfere with digestion and absorption.

- People who consume less animal protein have greater rates of bone loss than those who eat larger amounts of animal protein.

I will highlight the main animal protein sources below, and will comment about soy products and protein powders.

The Incredible, Edible Egg

Eggs are not just incredible, but what I would call the perfect food all wrapped up in one single cell. Yes, that's right, an egg is an individual cell, and contains the most complete and highest protein rating of any food, including all amino acids. Two eggs contain more than 12 grams of protein, just over half in the white and the rest in the yolk. In addition, eggs also contain many essential nutrients, including significant amounts of vitamins A, D, E, B1, B2, B6, folic acid and especially vitamin B12. Eggs also contain important minerals including calcium, magnesium, potassium, zinc and iron. Choline and biotin, also important for energy production and stress management, are contained in large amounts in eggs. Most of these nutrients are found in the yolk of the egg.

The fat in egg yolks is also nearly a perfect balance, containing mostly monounsaturated fats, and about 36 percent saturated fat. And, egg yolks contain linoleic and linolenic acids — both essential fatty acids. Eggs have almost no carbohydrate (less than 1 gram),

Some Facts about Eggs

The taming of chickens and other fowl for egg production dates back to before 1500 B.C. in China. Today, eggs come in many sizes and shell colors, not just white and brown. Depending on the type of chicken that laid them, some eggs have tints of green, blue and red.

Eggs, of course, should always be stored in the refrigerator. Because of their porous shell, there is slight evaporation of moisture from the inner egg through the shell, which changes its flavor and freshness. If you are not using them quickly, store your eggs in a sealed container to prevent loss of moisture. Never store eggs next to highly flavored foods, such as onions and fish, because they will easily absorb odors from these foods. Always store eggs with the large side up, which suspends the yolk effectively within the egg white.

Chefs know that room-temperature eggs are easier to work with; when boiled, they don't crack, the whites are easier to whip, and the yolks "stand up" more when fried. If you're separating eggs, however, the colder ones are easier to work with.

Speaking of boiled eggs, they should never really be boiled but kept just at a slight simmer until done. Furiously boiling them results in rubbery whites and less-tasty yolks. One way to prevent the shells from breaking during boiling is to use a pin. Prick the shell on the large end of the egg with a pin. This allows the air pocket, found in the large end of the egg, to escape during cooking. Otherwise, if the air can't escape, the pressure builds and it may crack the shell. The best way to cook soft- or hard-boiled eggs is to place them in cold water (1/2-inch above the eggs) and bring to a boil. Take off the heat immediately. For soft-cooked eggs, remove after 2-4 minutes, depending on your taste, and run under cold water. For hard-cooked eggs, cover and let sit for 15 minutes, then rinse in cold water and keep refrigerated until ready to use. (An egg that is less than two days old is very difficult to peel when hard-boiled.)

Finally, before you buy eggs make sure they are relatively fresh by looking at the date. Or, you can shake them close to your ear; if you hear a sloshing sound, it means they've lost a lot of moisture over time and there's a big air space in them — avoid these. Eggs also contain a natural barrier — an invisible protective coating that keeps out bacteria. Never wash eggs before storing because you will remove this natural protection.

making them the perfect meal or snack for the millions who are carbohydrate intolerant. Ounce per ounce, eggs are also your best food buy with hardly any waste. And, with so many ways of preparing them, eggs are delicious. While most people love the taste of eggs, many are still concerned about eating them because of cholesterol. For most people, eggs can be part of a healthy food plan. I eat several whole eggs every day. In the chapter on heart disease I'll address the issue of cholesterol, and how adding more eggs to your diet can actually decrease your cardiovascular risk.

Eggs are only as healthy as the hens that lay them, since the nutritional make-up of eggs, especially the fat, depends upon what the chickens eat. For this reason you should avoid run-of-the-mill grocery-store eggs that have been produced in chicken factories. Unfortunately this includes most eggs on the market. The healthiest eggs come from organic, free-range hens. Even better; buy eggs from a local farmer who lets chickens eat healthy, wild food and organic feed. Free-range means that the hens are allowed to roam where they can eat bugs and vegetable matter, yielding eggs with a better fat profile, with more monounsaturated fat and more essential fatty acids. So-called "omega 3" eggs come from chickens fed flaxseeds. Often these hens are not free-range nor certified organic and are still housed in very crowded hen factories.

Here's the Beef

It's no bull — if you want to be healthy, beef really is "what's for dinner." Consider that just 3 ounces of lean porterhouse contains 20 grams of protein, and just 6 grams of saturated fat, balanced by a healthy 7 grams of heart-friendly monounsaturated fat. In addition to being an excellent source of high-quality protein, beef is also rich in B vitamins, glutamine, calcium, magnesium, iron, zinc and other vital nutrients. Organic and natural beef have not been treated with antibiotics or given growth-stimulating hormones.

You can buy naturally raised meats in some grocery and health-food stores, and local sources may be even better. Look for nearby farms and ranches that sell meat from animals that have been raised on grass, not fed corn and without the use of growth hormones, antibiotics and other chemicals used by most stock-growers. Whether you live near a farm that sells natural or organic meat, or order from a ranch that can ship to you, you may wish to save money and buy a large quantity of beef so that you always have some on hand. The meat will keep well in a freezer until it's time to make another order.

When cooking beef, keep it on the rare side. Studies show that beef cooked medium, medium well, or well done is associated with higher rates of stomach cancer. This is due to the production of carcinogens (certain nitrogen compounds) created during cooking. Heat-sensitive nutrients, such as the amino acid glutamine, are also significantly reduced in meat cooked beyond rare. The less cooked the better. Bacteria in beef is usually due to the food-handling process. While bacteria can reside on the surface of meat, it won't get inside unless the meat is ground. Almost all cases of food poisoning involving meat are from sources that have been ground ahead of time. For this reason, ground meat should be thoroughly cooked unless it's freshly ground just before eating it.

The Poultry Flap

I rate eggs and beef as the best sources of protein but give poultry a poor rating due to how most of these animals are raised and processed. If you find an excellent source of chicken and turkey, and you really enjoy eating it, these are great protein foods.

The poultry industry has done such a good job telling you on paper how healthy chicken is over other meats, but this is untrue. In fact, because of lower standards, chickens are generally raised in more unhealthy environments than cattle and other animals. Today's chicken house is really an overpopulated filthy city, containing 100,000 birds or more, cooped up in tiny boxes or very crowded conditions. Because of this, most chickens are given many chemicals and drugs to counter common diseases and infections.

The best birds for the table are organically raised — they've not been treated with or fed any chemicals or drugs; instead, they are given certified-organic feeds and filtered water. This may be the safest of all poultry. Many grocery stores and health-food stores carry organic chickens and turkeys. In addition, you may be able to find birds such as these from a local farm.

The Catch to Fish

Fish can also be a great source of protein and some contain significant quantities of essential fatty acids, especially omega-3 fats. However, just as with other protein foods, some fish are healthier choices over others. The best sources are wild fish, not farm-raised.

In general, avoid seafood that includes the so-called bottom feeders, those fish and other sea species that eat from the ocean's floor, where the potential for consuming toxic material is highest. This is especially true for those species that feed close to shore. Flounder, sole, catfish and crab are some examples of foods to avoid eating regularly. Oysters, clams, mussels and scallops are also sources of potential pollutants. Clams are perhaps the worst seafood to eat, especially when raw, since they normally filter out and concentrate viruses and bacteria, heavy metals and other chemical pollutants from the waters in which they live. If you enjoy eating seafood, here are some tips for doing so more safely and more nutritiously:

- Choose fish caught in waters farther away from polluted, industrial areas. Some examples are Canadian salmon, sardines and herring.

- Look for cold-water fish like salmon, dark tuna, sardines and other small fish that contain higher amounts of omega-3 fat and EPA.

- Eat smaller fish and crustaceans: trout, bass and shrimp and avoid marlin, white tuna and swordfish. Smaller and younger fish have not accumulated the toxins found in larger fish and older species.

- Limit your intake of shellfish, and choose smaller species such as smaller shrimp.

- Avoid precooked fish, and prepared or processed seafood such as breaded fish or seafood, fish cakes, ground fish and imitation crabmeat.

- If you catch your own fish, ask local authorities about the limits of safety. Some regions recommend limiting how much of certain species you should eat in a year.

Unfortunately, the oceans, rivers and lakes are becoming so contaminated that wild fish are containing levels of toxins that are dangerous. I recommend limiting fish to once or twice a month or less, and even less than that for children and pregnant women.

The picture is worse for farm-raised seafood — this should always be avoided. These foods often include antibiotics, pesticides, steroids, hormones and artificial pigments. Unfortunately, they are becoming popular due to availability and cost. For example, farm-raised salmon makes up 95 percent of the salmon on the market today. Since these fish are raised in confined, crowded and unsanitary conditions, the threat of disease and parasites is great. To combat disease and parasites, some fish farmers add antibiotics to salmon feed, and treat the salmon and their pens with pesticides. Some fish are also treated with steroids to make the fish sterile, and growth hormones to speed them to market size and reduce production costs. In addition, since farm-raised salmon do not naturally eat crustaceans that naturally make the flesh pink or orange, salmon growers often feed color additives to pigment the flesh.

Other Meaty Matters

In addition to beef, poultry and fish, other meats are also good sources of protein. Pork and lamb are popular meats, and recently meats such as buffalo and elk have appeared in some groceries. When choosing these meats use the same guidelines as with beef and poultry — buy those that are organic or raised naturally at a local farm.

Wild game, including big-game animals such as deer as well as small game such as rabbits and game birds, is also another great source of protein. Wild-game meat is generally leaner but higher in essential fatty acids than domestic meats. While hunting your own meat is nearly ideal, there is a growing concern in some areas like the northeastern United States that the use of pesticides and other environmental chemicals has affected wild animals. But in general, wild game is much safer than store-bought meat.

Generally avoid ground meat of any kind unless it has been freshly ground right before deep freezing or eating it. Ground meat is a haven for bacteria and can ferment in your intestine much worse than whole meat. If you like ground meat or have a recipe that requires it, it's best to buy a large piece of meat and then grind it up just before cooking — most butchers, even those in large groceries, will do this for you. Also beware of other meats that have already been cut, such as sliced meat, chopped meat and stew meat. Try to buy as large a piece of meat as possible and cut it yourself.

Processed meats can also be unhealthy choices. Most sausage, lunch meats and other processed meats are not only ground, but also may contain high amounts of sugar and chemicals that you don't want to eat. However, it is possible to find organic bacon and hams that have been cured with honey and with no harmful chemicals.

The most nutritious parts of the animal to eat are the organs and glands. In our society, the liver is the most common organ food, with stomach, brains, kidneys and others only rarely eaten. However, when a lion kills his prey, it's the organs and glands that are first devoured. The muscle, what we refer to as the "meat," is often left for the scavengers. Unfortunately, with our polluted environment, organ meats such as liver are becoming more dangerous since it's the liver's job to filter the blood and remove toxins from the body. If you enjoy liver and other organ and gland meats, be sure to find a very good source.

Say Cheese!

Cheese and plain yogurt are dairy products that contain quality protein without many of the problems associated with milk. This is especially true if you can find organic products made from raw milk. Also consider that goat and sheep milk are much more compatible for humans than cow milk. These cheeses can be found in many stores and on the Internet.

Whichever type of milk they're made from, cultured products such as cheese and yogurt are good sources of complete protein with the lactose, or "milk sugar" reduced by friendly bacteria in the culturing process. To be sure that an item is fully cultured, check the "Nutrition Facts" on the label; the carbohydrate should be very low. (Of course you want to avoid the fruit-flavored and sweetened varieties of yogurt that are always full of sugar — sometimes a half-dozen teaspoons or more!)

It's important to remember that dairy is also high in B fat. So you must be careful to eat cheese in a way that maintains balance with your intake of A and C fats. If you are recovering from an inflammatory-related illness, such as cancer, heart disease and the others discussed in this book, limit or avoid dairy products. In addition, avoid so-called "American" cheese, cheese spreads and other processed cheeses. These highly processed products, which outsell natural cheese, are usually several types of unripe cheeses, ground up with added chemical stabilizers, preservatives and emulsifiers.

Curds and Whey

Remember Little Miss Muffet, eating her curds and whey? These are the two proteins found in milk. Whey protein is the thin liquid part of milk remaining after the casein (the curds) and fat are removed. Whey is the part of the milk containing most of the vitamins and minerals, including calcium, and it's a complete protein. During the making of cheese, which mostly is produced from curds, whey is often fed back to the animals for nutritional reasons.

The whey component of milk contains a group of natural sulfur-containing substances called biothiols that help produce a key antioxidant in your cells (called glutathione). Because it helps the immune system, whey has been used to help prevent and treat many chronic conditions, from asthma and allergies to cancer and heart disease. It can also help improve muscle function. Most people who are allergic to cow's milk can usually consume whey without problems. Small amounts of lactose are found in whey (much less than is found in liquid milk) but this is usually too little to cause intestinal problems, even in most people sensitive to lactose. In those who are truly lactose-intolerant (probably less than 5 percent of the population), this amount of lactose could be a problem.

Most cheeses are made from curds, but some are made from whey. Italian ricotta is the most common one; check the ingredient label on ricotta to make sure the main ingredient is whey. Whey is also made into powders for use in baked goods and smoothies as discussed below.

The curds from milk are used for most cheese making. Cottage cheese is the best example of what curds look like. However, the curd is the protein in milk most people are allergic to when there's a dairy allergy. Newborns and young children are especially vulnerable to curds because their intestines and immune systems are too immature to tolerate this protein.

The Soy Story

While soy is a vegetarian source of a complete protein, it's often a problem for most people. One reason is that most soy in use today is highly processed and concentrated. Whole green soybeans or edamame are an example of a whole food, and a good source of protein. With a relatively small amount of simple processing soy can be made into tofu, also a good food. This is how most soy has been consumed for many years, and studies of these populations seem to show that soy has health benefits when consumed as a food.

But most soy today highly processed and concentrated. For example, many soy powders used in food products and supplements are so concentrated that a serving or two would be like eating a pound or more of real soybeans — something most people would never even consider. For this reason, it's best to avoid all processed soy products, including soy-protein isolates and caseinates and hydrolyzed soy. The more soy is processed, the worse it can be. Monosodium glutamate (MSG), a one-time commonly used powder that makes food seemingly taste better (still used in Chinese and other restaurants) is made by processing soy. So products containing isolated or hydrolyzed soy also include some MSG (but it is not required to be listed in the ingredients).

Many people, especially children, may be intolerant and even allergic to soy in all forms. In addition concentrated soy isoflavones, used in dietary supplements can pose serious dangers, including hormonal imbalance, which can increase the risk of cancer, particularly for post-menopausal women, the very audience these products are marketed to by the big companies.

Protein Powders

Soy, milk, whey, egg and other foods are commonly sold to supplement the diet. These have value when used cautiously. Certainly avoid any of these powders if you're intolerant to those foods. In addition, avoid all powders that have been isolated, caseinated or hydrolyzed. These products are touted as being highest in protein — which is true, but at the expense of being highly processed and containing MSG. Those marked "concentrated" are the least processed of the powders and are an acceptable part of a healthy diet. Egg white powder is the least processed of all the powders. This and whey concentrate are the best and healthiest of all these products. (If you use egg white powder in a blender, you must include a small amount of fat otherwise it will create a large volume of foam — great for meringue but not for smoothies and other recipes.)

Most importantly, when choosing protein sources look for real food. Fresh whole eggs, whole pieces of meat and fish, raw-milk cheese as tolerated. Avoid the processed protein products — cold cuts, frozen foods, processed cheese, etc. If you need to increase protein intake with a food supplement, use egg white powder or a whey concentrate. These foods also contain a variety of important vitamins, minerals and phytonutrients. Another key food group — which complements these protein foods rather well — are vegetables, the topic of the next chapter.

13

Vital Vegetables and Fruits

So far we've looked in depth at the three macronutrients — carbohydrate, proteins and fats — as the basis of good nutrition. Now let's shift gears and take a look at a group of foods that really should have their own distinct classification — vegetables and fruits. Plant foods should make up the bulk of your dietary intake because they contain vitamins, minerals and, just as important, phytonutrients. And, there are thousands of phytonutrients that scientists believe may have an even more important role than vitamins in promoting health and preventing disease. Fruits and vegetables also contain small amounts of protein and essential fatty acids, and are a key source of fiber and prebiotics, which are both essential for good health, as we will learn in the following chapter.

Generally fruits are foods that contain a seed within, whereas vegetables have a separate seed. Both contain some carbohydrates, some high enough for those who are carbohydrate intolerant to avoid. These include most potatoes, corn, watermelon, pineapple and dried fruits.

Some foods that are technically fruits are usually thought of as vegetables — these include avocados, tomatoes, eggplant, peppers, squash and other fruits that are not sweet. But basically, vegetables and fruits are all plant foods that should make up the bulk of the diet. Most people don't eat enough vegetables and fruits, and there are very, very few who eat too much of this good thing. I often recommend as a general guideline that people try to eat at least 10 servings of vegetables and fruits per day. Many of these should be raw, and most, if not all, should be fresh.

What is a serving? Traditionally many have considered a serving to be a half-cup. More recently, however, many dietary guidelines have recommended different approaches for measuring servings. For instance, a serving of lettuce might be a cup and a half; a serving of carrots might be one medium carrot; a serving of broccoli is one medium stalk, and a serving of asparagus is five spears. Using guidelines like these will help you to eat more vegetables than using the traditional half-cup serving.

Vegetables: The Main Course

Many people think of vegetables as a tedious side dish. But it's best to consider vegetables part of a main dish. This may require adjusting the way you think about your meals. Think first what your main-course vegetable will be, and then make your other foods the side dishes — usually some sort of protein or an unrefined carbohydrate. In this way you can make vegetables the bulk of your diet. Experiment in creating other types of meals around vegetables. For instance a vegetable omelet with onions, red and yellow peppers and zucchini makes a meal out of eggs at breakfast. A vegetable-based organic-chicken soup with garlic, leeks, carrots, celery, and even green beans and yellow squash, is a bowl full of nutrition for lunch. Even Mom's meat loaf can be adjusted to include half vegetables — start with chopped onions, red or yellow bell peppers, zucchini, fresh parsley and garlic, and then add freshly chopped meat and at least two whole eggs, and season with sea salt and spices of your choice.

In choosing your vegetables don't overlook cooked greens. Some of the most neglected vegetables, such as kale, mustard greens, rapini, Swiss chard, collards and the common spinach, are also some of the most nutritious. These bitter leafy vegetables are full of valuable phytonutrients, as well as a host of vitamins and minerals. Once you get used to the idea of cooking greens, some meals just won't seem complete without them — truly, cooked greens can be served as a delicious bed for just about any protein food, from beef to fish. Greens can simply be steamed and served with a little butter or extra-virgin olive oil and sea salt. Or, add other vegetables to the mix, such as leeks, chopped white onions, mushrooms or red and yellow peppers. Cook your greens until they are slightly tender, but be careful not to overcook, lest you lose the vital nutrients. Just when they turn bright green is about right.

Choose a Rainbow of Colors

In addition to eating enough vegetables it is important to eat a variety of these foods as well. The reason is that different vegetables contain varying amounts of specific nutrients. For instance a serving of leaf lettuce supplies a high amount of beta carotene but only a small amount of vitamin C, while a serving of Brussels sprouts contains high levels of vitamin C with a small amount of beta carotene.

One of the easiest ways to ensure that you eat enough variety in vegetables is to use the "rainbow" technique. Choosing vegetables in a rainbow of colors will help ensure a variety of nutrients. For example, carrots and winter squash, which are orange, are high in beta carotene, which is converted by the body to vitamin A. Many green vegetables are high in vitamin C — a serving of broccoli, for example, is very high in vitamin C. In addition to orange and green vegetables, consider purple eggplant and cabbage, red peppers, white, green and red onions, white cauliflower, yellow summer squash, brown mushrooms and many others. Each of these colorful vegetables contains its own unique set of vitamins, minerals and phytonutrients.

A Salad a Day

In reaching your goal of 10 servings of vegetables and fruits per day, it's important to make sure much of this is raw. In fact, each meal should contain some raw food. Salads, large and small, can easily provide this raw food. Your salad can be a snack, a side dish or, with some added protein, it can be a meal in itself. Salad is a low-stress food, with no cooking involved and minimal cleanup. The base for a great salad, of course, is something green — fresh lettuce, spinach or even young kale. Buy organic and buy often, but avoid iceberg lettuce as it has one of the lowest overall nutritional values of all vegetables. The little bags of baby greens are fine so long as you eat them quickly. You can also buy whole heads of green- or red-leaf, Romaine, Bibb and endive lettuces. Then, for a few days of really quick salads, clean a whole head of lettuce, dry the leaves well (spinning works great) and refrigerate them in an airtight container with a piece of paper towel. Your lettuce will be ready to go when you need it.

Use a variety of raw vegetables such as carrots, chopped red and yellow peppers, purple cabbage, tomatoes and avocados. Separately, these can be used for meals that don't contain a salad. In addition, steamed and chilled green beans and asparagus also liven up a salad. Chopped walnuts, slivered almonds, piñon nuts, gourmet olives, capers and artichoke hearts make a salad even more exotic.

To make your salad into a true meal, add some protein. Lightly grilled tuna, wild shrimp, sliced beefsteak, hard-boiled eggs or shredded goat cheese are some options. Of course, a great salad requires a delicious dressing. My healthy salad dressing is great (recipe follows), but simple extra-virgin olive oil and vinegar is fine too. Always use your own homemade dressing and avoid the additives that come out of a bottle.

The best way to add fruits to your diet, including berries, is to use them as they are — as a snack, a healthy dessert, or made into recipes such as smoothies. Some of these are discussed in the chapter on snacks. Fruits are also a delicious part of a salad; for example, an arugula salad with sliced pears and goat cheese, or an apple walnut salad with greens.

Phil's Healthy Salad Dressing

Mix in a glass jar with tight-fitting lid:

- 8 ounces extra-virgin olive oil
- 2 cloves finely chopped garlic
- 2 ounces or more apple-cider vinegar
- 1 tablespoon fresh or dried parsley
- 2 teaspoons sea salt
- 1/2 teaspoon mustard

Option: Add 1 to 2 tablespoons plain yogurt, or sour cream.
Use other good-quality oils for variations in taste.
Shake well before serving. Refrigerate.

The Bitter Truth

It's now clear that naturally occurring substances known as phytonutrients, or phytochemicals, found in vegetables and fruits, may be more important to good nutrition than vitamins and can help prevent and treat cancer and other diseases. Their actions halt the production of cancer-causing agents in the body, blocking activation of these chemicals, or suppressing the spread of cancer cells that already exist. The vegetables and fruits researchers think are most capable of preventing cancer and other diseases, including heart disease, are green leafy vegetables, broccoli, Brussels sprouts, cabbage, onions, citrus fruit (not the juice), grapes, red wine, green tea and others. The more bitter, the better.

How many times have you heard that if something tastes good then it must not be good for you, or vice-versa? While this is a gross generalization, many people avoid eating bitter-tasting vegetables and fruits, which are particularly high in the natural disease-preventing phytonutrients that cause their bitterness. In general, the more bitter the taste, the more rich the food is in these phytonutrients.

For plants, these bitter-tasting substances — the healthy phytonutrients — serve as natural insect repellents and pesticides. Some are even toxic to small animals like birds, mice and rats, including some compounds in cabbage and Brussels sprouts. Generally, higher amounts of bitter-tasting phytonutrients are found in sprouts and seedlings than in mature plants. This provides young plants with a type of natural protection from being eaten at an early stage of life, before the chance of reproduction. But you would have to consume pounds and pounds of vegetables daily to ingest toxic amounts of phytonutrients.

Despite the therapeutic and nutritive value of phytonutrients, the food industry is solving the so-called "problem" of bitterness in fruits and vegetables by removing these healthful chemicals through genetic engineering and selective breeding. Unfortunately, our culture has associated bitterness with bad taste instead of health promotion. Now many agricultural scientists, who want foods sweeter, are changing our food supply for us — they are literally removing the healthy components from certain foods in order to sell more food products. And they are succeeding. Canola oil, for example, contains significant reductions of phytonutrients due to selective breeding. And transgenic citrus is now a reality — it's sweeter, but it's also free of limonene, the bitter substance that can help prevent and treat skin cancer.

Cancer researchers propose that a heightened sense of bitterness might be a healthy trait, allowing people to select foods with the highest phytonutrient content. This view contrasts with the food industry's practice of measuring the content of these bitter phytonutrients merely as a way of developing new non-bitter, phytonutrient-deficient strains. So while some nutrition scientists propose enhancing phytonutrients in foods for better health, the standard industry practice has been to remove them for better taste. Indeed, the lower amount of bitter compounds in the modern diet reflects the "achievement" of the food industry. The irony is that as agricultural scientists remove more phytonutrients from plants, farmers have to use even more chemical pesticides to protect their crops; thus consumers are left with the double-whammy of vegetables and fruits with less nutrition and more harmful pesticides.

In addition to bitterness, an astringent taste is also associated with healthy phytonutrients. These tastes can actually be quite attractive. Consider a fine aged Bordeaux wine or a high-quality green tea. Unfortunately, these are exceptions and sweetness is a dominant taste preference, or perhaps "addiction" is a better word.

You can get more phytonutrients into your diet by eating foods that have a natural bitter or astringent taste. Zucchini and other squashes, pumpkins, cucumbers, melon, citrus and many other vegetables and fruits, along with almonds and many types of beans, contain natural phytonutrients, as do red wine, green tea and cocoa.

Eat as much of as many types of vegetables and fruits as you can, both cooked and raw. Making these healthy vegetable choices is just another journey on the road to optimal health and human performance. In addition to variety, the highest quality vegetables and fruits may be those that are organically grown, as discussed in the next chapter.

14

Organic Foods

Today's consumers may find a large variety of certified-organic produce, meats and other foods in traditional "health food" stores, and now even in conventional grocery stores. Two common questions are whether it's worth the extra price to buy organic food versus conventional, and whether we can trust the sign that says "certified organic."

With great hesitation my answer to both questions is yes, but with an asterisk. The USDA organic program is now part of an international phenomenon. The regulations are better than the previous unregulated organic movement, when anyone could say a product was organic. Many of the guidelines are potentially good for consumers — organic animals must be raised with organic feed, filtered water and certified organic pastures, and many commonly used drugs can't be used. Organic produce must be grown without commonly used pesticides, herbicides and other chemicals. Many food product ingredients — additives, chemicals, preservatives and others are not allowed in organic foods. And, the program is relatively strict, helping to rid the market of dishonest vendors. So if a product has the USDA organic label, it's as good as the USDA's ability to police the program, just like the rest of what the agency does for all foods sold to consumers. But like the rest of our food supply, you have to be a careful consumer, reading labels and being aware of and avoiding organic junk food, which makes up most of today's organic products.

True to Jerome Irving Rodale's ideas of the mid 1900s, organic food is better, whether certified or not. For example, organic vegetables and fruits usually taste better. They've not been genetically altered, and contain much smaller amounts of chemical fertilizers, or none at all. Moreover, many studies indicate that organic produce is more nutritious, containing more vitamins, minerals and phytonutrients. Some of the nutrients studied in organic produce were twice that of conventional equivalents. Many vegetables have been studied, including carrots, cabbage, lettuce, kale, tomatoes and spinach, with a variety of fruits studied by various researchers. The increased nutrients found in certified-organic vegetables and fruits are most likely due to better care of the soil through organic farming methods, including composting, crop rotation and cover crops.

I've also conducted my own research and found that some organically grown vegetables had significantly higher levels — 10 times or more — of certain nutrients such as folic acid, compared to the same vegetables tested and listed in the USDA database.

For years, nutritionists insisted that today's conventionally grown foods were as high in vitamins and minerals as the meals of our grandparents. There is now sufficient evidence indicating this is not necessarily the case. Reductions in food quality have taken place since the mid-1940s, when the use of chemical fertilizers and pesticides rapidly became the norm in U.S. farming. A study in the *British Food Journal* compared the 1930s nutrient content of 20 fruits and vegetables with foods grown in the 1980s. Significant reductions were found in the levels of calcium, copper and magnesium in vegetables; and magnesium, iron, copper and potassium in fruit. Similar trends can be found in foods produced in the United States, with reductions in some nutrients of as much as 30 percent.

Most foods are farmed with chemical fertilizers and pesticides, with the exception of certified organic foods, which contain significantly less nitrates and heavy metals, both of which can be very harmful, especially to children. Heavy metals enter the plants through certain chemical fertilizers — some of these fertilizers are even derived from industrial waste. As discussed earlier, important phytonutrients have been genetically engineered out of some common foods to make them less bitter. Organically grown foods don't contain genetically engineered ingredients or genetically modified organisms, making them a better choice.

Then there's another factor to consider when choosing organic food. Many of the foods in grocery stores are imported. The countries of origin may not have as stringent restrictions regarding the use of fertilizers and especially pesticides as we have in this country. In fact, some countries still allow the use of pesticides that were banned decades ago in the United States. Choosing organic produce eliminates this potential problem.

When shopping for organic food, watch out for the organic junk food — it's all over the store! Buy the basics — real food. This includes vegetables, fruits, meats, nuts, seeds, cheese and eggs.

Buy Local?

With the problems in the organic industry, including the dilution of a strict standard in growing and producing the cleanest and highest quality foods, and the added costs due to the certification process, many truly health-conscious consumers once again are looking for healthy options. They're seeing the potential of the traditional farmer's markets, community organic cooperatives, roadside farm stands, and "pick-your-own" programs. Internet shopping for organic food is growing, especially in bulk quantity. These modern markets feature products grown in a "green" way — produced in line with the original organic movement despite having the name taken away by the USDA and other agencies worldwide. And, they often include a "buy local" slogan.

The problem is there is no regulation regarding whether it's "green," organic or beyond organic. One result is that, in some cases, authorities have stopped farmers from selling their products. Another problem is the notion that products that are better than organic — the "beyond organic" movement — should be more expensive. But just because products are grown with care, without chemicals, doesn't mean they should be more expensive. Without the "middlemen" — typically two, three or more of them taking a share before products get to the retail stores, most of these products should be less expensive than the same or similar products in retail stores.

Despite these issues, if you're a careful consumer and talk to the farmers and those producing these products, and even visit their farms, you can usually find high-quality healthy products that are often better than the organic versions in retail stores, often for less cost. Supply and demand will help weed out the overpriced products.

Virtually all the food I buy is organic, although more and more is not USDA-certified organic. And I buy the basics — vegetables, fruits, meat, eggs, cheese, nuts and seeds. The most impressive operation I've seen is the Double Check Ranch in central Arizona, where I buy all my beef. While they don't participate in the national organic program, I have inspected their ranch and would certify them as "beyond organic." This ranch is clean, efficient, inspected by local government, and has a philosophy of not just producing healthy food, but incorporates an approach to farming that's good for the land as well. (Their website provides many informative articles — www.DoubleCheckRanch.com.)

I buy fresh eggs from a local producer that's not certified organic, but the eggs are better than the ones that are certified. I also buy food from local farmer's markets if I know the food is from a good source. And I have bulk items shipped. Most of these foods are cheaper than the organic versions in the retail stores. And, my large garden provides a significant amount of food that is also "beyond organic."

The Organic Movement

We're not sure just when the organic movement started. That would depend, in part, on how you define it. Certainly in the early stages, the word "organic" was not part of it. This word would not be introduced until around 1941 by a British chemist Sir Albert Howard. But by then, the movement was decades old and had more than one front. There were those who promoted the scientific reasons for farming with a natural process; those who had more spiritual reasons to care for the land; small farmers who were being left out of big business; those with strong social attitudes who wanted to help the "little guys" get a fair share of the profits; and consumers, who eventually had the greatest numbers and created the real change. But even before the movement was noticed, there were those few who made the observations that growing food in the most natural soils produced better food and healthier people.

In the 1830s German chemist Justus von Liebig was formulating his agricultural biochemistry theories, which he published in the 1840s, discussing how plants utilize nitrogen in the soil along with various minerals. Natural fertilizers, he theorized, including manure, would provide these nutrients. This was the beginning of modern farming, and the movement soon branched into two: One became big business farming, with newly developing chemical fertilizers and pesticides, and the other was the organic movement. Sir Albert Howard may be one of the earliest "organic" farmers — he was from a British farming family but learned about natural soil production and organic gardening in India in 1905.

With the influence of Howard's writings — he called the introduction of chemical fertilizers and pesticides a great threat to the future of human health — there was a clear separation of the organic movement and conventional farming. His writing spread throughout Europe and eventually to America.

By the early 1900s, American food manufacturers, as an integral part of the "modern farming" movement, began mass-producing the first packaged foods. This coincided with a major change from the farmer's markets with its many single food stands, to one store that would sell all types of food — a "super market" — complete with the latest technology of packaged foods. Small groups of concerned citizens immediately and openly protested against the mass packaging of food. Some, including Dr. Royal Lee, began growing high quality food with natural composting, and in 1929 he began manufacturing the first dietary supplements in America using these foods.

By the 1930s, with the influence of Howard's writings and others in America, the organic movement was organized, albeit small. One person who jumped on board was an engineer named Jerome Irving Rodale. He not only bought a farm and began organic gardening but started publishing a magazine on organic methods in the 1940s — and Sir Albert Howard would contribute articles. Rodale also started a printing business that would also publish books — a business that thrives today as a multi-million-dollar corporation.

I was introduced to Rodale's books on organic gardening in the 1960s, and soon after planted my first organic garden. As a student working part time in a health-food store, and, having studied basic chemistry, I realized almost all the vitamins on the shelves were synthetic, not natural as they claimed. Seeing a growing market in the organic industry, the pharmaceutical companies had quietly jumped on board by producing virtually all the synthetic vitamins for the health food industry, a problem that continues today.

After studying organic gardening and natural health, and many different health-care philosophies, I decided to go back to college, become a doctor and focus on helping people get healthy.

Into the 1970s and '80s, the organic movement continued to hold its social, fair trade and health-oriented subgroups. Even up to the time when the USDA decided to take charge of the movement by creating a National Organic Program (NOP) in 1990 that would define organic and certify growers, manufacturers and others involved in the organic movement, there continued to be different philosophies associated with organics.

The NOP would spend the next decade gathering information from the organic movement, create standards, rules, regulations and a system to certify all those it would allow into the organic movement — often for a hefty price — under the guise that the USDA needed to regulate the process. The result was the "certified organic" regulations, released in 2002, complete with a seal of authenticity. USDA established three levels of organic: 100 percent, 95 percent, which allowed 5 percent non-organic material, and 70 percent organic.

There was one problem: During this decade big business lobbied heavily for regulations that would make it easier and cheaper to jump on the "certified organic" bandwagon. Not only that, the large manufacturers of processed foods, the sugar industry, large food chains and a variety of other lobbyists made sure they were part of the process. The result was a massive growth of organic junk food that coincided with the NOP's "organic" launch in 2002.

Just before the NOP became law, I created, in 1999, the first line of certified-organic dietary supplements made from real food. I followed the developments of the USDA's certified organic program and prepared my formulas based on what I thought would be the requirements for organic certification. These were easily met, and today, these dietary supplements are sold by First Organics, Inc.

The Organic Trade Association (OTA) evolved from part of the movement that was the political tail. Its goal was to help companies involved in certified organic activities work with other companies and the NOP. Unfortunately, it was a political organization not oriented to health. At its first national trade show, I was shocked at the number of organic junk food companies represented — you could sample organic cookies made from organic white flour and organic white sugar, eat processed organic corn chips, drink organic beer, and even smoke organic cigarettes. This was the modern health food industry! But the worst was yet to come.

There were a number of speakers discussing the value of organic certification. A keynote speaker was JI Rodale's granddaughter, who was a main player in the Rodale publishing empire. She was so excited to see the organic movement get this far and be so successful. After her talk, she took questions. I asked, "Are you concerned that the organic industry is made up of so much junk food that adversely affects people's health?" Her answer was an emphatic no. She said that people can make their own choices.

Marie Rodale's grandfather, JI, promoted the relationship between organic farming and optimal health, and helped launch the organic movement. But now, companies making organic junk food have become the biggest advertising revenue for the modern Rodale publishing empire. In joining with big business and the USDA, the small farmers and start-up companies making healthy foods were left out.

Meanwhile, consumers jumped in too. They were the ones eating all the organic junk food. This was evident just by looking — at the owners, employees and others working in the "health food" industry, including those in the stores. Go into Whole Foods, for example, and you'll see the shelves full of organic junk. And a large part of the store is the bakery section — complete with white flour and sugar cakes, cookies and pies.

My level of disappointment in the organic movement has reached a high. My first article after returning home from the OTA show, "organic junk," brought praise by a few but anger from industry people. Making money, it seemed, was the goal of certified organics, even if it contributed to the explosion of obesity not only in adults, but young children. Along the way, the large companies, including manufacturers and grocery stores, along with the two "new" health food chains, successfully pushed for the NOP regulations to be diluted — many unhealthy foods, food additives and other ingredients would now be allowed in organic foods. I began writing and lecturing more on the dangers of organic junk food, and "beyond organic" — those small farmers, companies and consumers left out of the original organic movement who were still there hoping for healthy changes. The organic movement had left them behind. And many legitimate farmers, manufacturers and food companies that were too small to pay the thousands of dollars to be part of the USDA's organic movement were actually creating healthier food.

Where are we now? At the time of this writing, early in 2009, I'm very disillusioned with the government-sponsored organic programs. And because the USDA took the word "organic" for itself, products or companies would not be allowed to use the word "organic" unless it was certified by the USDA. In addition, small farms, legitimate companies producing healthy foods and others involved in the organic movement are even being harassed by federal and local authorities because they have not embraced the movement. The result is that a small but growing movement continues, made up of consumers and health-care professionals like me, seeking the best food from good and honest people all working together for a healthier planet.

If you really want the highest-quality produce, the best option is to grow your own. If you have any yard space at all, a small vegetable plot, properly tended, can yield enough vegetables in season for your entire family. Many areas have community gardens, where many individuals share in a larger plot of land. By growing your own vegetables you can ensure their quality, reduce the price of your produce and revel in the enjoyment of producing your own food, not to mention the extra exercise you get from working in your garden.

15

The Full Spectrum of Fiber

Vegetables, fruits and other plant materials contain certain types of food particles that are not digestible or absorbable, but have powerful health-promoting effects. These include fiber and prebiotics; both improve function of the colon, a part of the large intestine, by promoting bulk growth of healthy bacteria. Fiber and prebiotics have a symbiotic relationship that not only promotes healthy colon activity but also is important to overall body function. Dietary fiber and prebiotics are found in vegetables, fruits, herbs and grains, and are the elements that give structure to the cell walls of these plant foods.

Fiber Foods

There are various types of fibers with different names, depending on the part of the plant and type of plant from which they are derived. By eating a variety of natural foods, you can obtain the full spectrum of these fibers. They include pectin, cellulose, beta-glucans, mucilages and a variety of gums including guar, arabic and locust bean.

Pectin is the substance partly responsible for the ripening of fruit. It is especially high in apples, citrus and most berries and is used as a gelling agent in foods such as jam. Applesauce is a high-pectin food that works as a remedy for diarrhea by adding bulk to the intestinal contents. Cellulose, such as found in wheat bran, is a component of cell walls of most plants. Beta-glucans from oats have become popular because of their positive association with reducing the risk of cardiovascular disease. Mucilages, such as psyllium and seaweed, are very functional fibers rich in minerals. Natural gums, as extracted from certain plants, have been used for thousands of years as thickening agents and emulsifiers, and can also benefit the intestine.

It's not so important to remember all the different names of these natural fibers. But it is important to remember to eat a variety of vegetables and fruits, which will provide you with the full spectrum of fiber important not only for your intestines but for your entire system. When, and if, you eat too much of one particular type of fiber, and consume it apart from those in natural foods, you risk creating an imbalance. It's analogous to the ABCs of fat — balance is the key. Try to get all the fiber you need by eating a variety of healthy food, especially vegetables and fruits. At least one, preferably two or even three, semi-solid bowel movements per day is a general indication that you're eating enough fiber.

If you still feel you need more fiber after eating adequate fiber-rich foods and drinking enough water, you can supplement your diet with additional concentrated sources. Different people respond differently to specific types of fiber, but generally the herb psyllium performs very well in most people. This is especially useful in those people who have reduced grains and other carbohydrate foods.

Physical Aspects of Fiber

Fiber, by definition, is not absorbable. This has certain specific and important implications for the intestines. First, fiber acts as a vehicle, helping to transport food through the intestines at a healthy rate. The more-rapid transit time that results from fiber in the diet also limits the amount of time cancer-causing chemicals are in contact with the intestine's cells. After the body absorbs whatever nutrients it can get from the non-fiber portion of the meal, that food (now referred to as waste) is eliminated via the large intestine with great assistance from fiber. In addition, fiber affects the viscosity of the food, beginning in the stomach, and controls the rate of digestion. Too little fiber results in a too-rapid digestion in the upper intestine.

Fiber also is capable of holding water in the intestine, which has an important function of diluting potential toxins, including carcinogens, and preventing constipation. These toxins may also attach to the fiber and be removed from the body.

In the large intestine, fiber provides the proper environment for the growth of "friendly" bacteria, which have a very important function. These micro-organisms ferment some of the fiber substances, improving the health of the intestine and other areas of metabolism. Intestinal bacteria also produce important fatty acids. These fats regulate the acid-alkaline balance in the large intestine and in turn control the bacteria themselves. Some fatty acids serve as an important energy source for the cells in the lower intestine. One specific fatty acid, butyric, may also play a protective role against cancer by maintaining a low colon pH and directly inhibiting tumor formation.

The process of fermentation also results in intestinal gas (mostly hydrogen and methane). If there's too much gas, causing discomfort or pain, it's a sign that there's a problem. Some of this gas is actually absorbed via the large intestine into the body, and is released through the lungs. Those individuals with bad breath usually have too much fermentation or gas from unfriendly bacteria. In any of these instances, stress, the wrong foods (typically too much carbohydrate) or too little fiber, among other problems, can be the cause. Antibiotic use, which kills the friendly microorganisms in the intestine, can also be a cause. This destruction of the normal bacteria results in a "re-colonization" of the large intestine with unfriendly bacteria. Yogurt, which contains friendly bacteria, can be helpful in these situations. Furthermore, eating foods that contain prebiotics helps promote the growth of healthy bacteria in the colon, as discussed later in this chapter.

The beneficial effects of fiber on bile (from the liver and gall bladder) may also help prevent intestinal cancers. Excess amounts of bile in the colon may cause normal cells to convert to cancerous ones. By eating enough fiber and enough variety of fiber, the concentration of bile in the colon remains lower.

Fiber and Absorption of Nutrients

Another important function of fiber is how it affects the absorption of nutrients from your diet. For example, fiber in your meal can slow sugar (glucose) absorption, and lower the glycemic index of that meal. Remember that the glycemic index is a measure of the blood-sugar response to certain foods or meals. Fiber-rich foods generally have a lower glycemic index and when consumed result in less insulin production. This makes fiber especially important for anyone with carbohydrate intolerance. Pectins, mucilages, and especially gums, seem to do this very well.

Absorption of minerals is also influenced by fiber, but in a negative way. Phytic acid, a natural substance present in the fibers of grains and in much smaller amounts in fruits, can inhibit the absorption of calcium, iron, zinc and copper, and possibly other nutrients. For those who may have problems getting enough of these minerals, limiting grains can be helpful.

In addition to their relationship to mineral absorption, some fibers may have an adverse effect on digestive enzymes. Wheat bran, for example, can inhibit the production of pancreatic enzymes responsible for digesting carbohydrates, proteins and fats. The fiber in legumes may inhibit the enzyme amylase, which is important for carbohydrate digestion. Other studies show that the fiber in many cereals contains pancreatic inhibitors that can diminish protein digestion. In addition, the fiber in unprocessed soybeans can induce an allergy-type reaction in some people, accounting for the intestinal discomfort some may have with soy.

Energy from Fiber

Since fiber is not absorbed, it does not directly count as an energy source. For this reason, if you eat a slice of whole-grain bread that contains 15 grams of carbohydrate, you really can't count it as 15 grams of usable energy, since some of that carbohydrate is fiber. If that slice of bread contains four grams of fiber, subtract four grams from the 15 grams of total carbohydrate, giving a total of 11 grams of usable carbohydrate.

While the fiber grams are not directly counted as energy calories, the body does indirectly obtain energy from fiber through fermentation by bacteria in the large intestine. As mentioned previously, fiber provides the environment for this bacterial activity. The bacteria produce short-chain fatty acids, typically butyric, acetic and propionic, which are absorbed and used by the body as fuel. Some fibers, such as pectin, are more capable of producing energy than others, such as fiber from grains. Approximately two calories of energy can be produced per gram of fiber. This is compared to four calories for other dietary carbohydrates, four for protein and nine for dietary fats.

Prebiotics — the Other 'Fiber'

Most of us have heard about the many benefits of dietary fiber, but certain fiber-like foods called prebiotics can even more dramatically improve the function and health of the colon. Prebiotics include one group of natural non-digestible carbohydrates called fructans. Fructan-rich foods should be eaten daily, if possible. Fructans are contained in small amounts in most plant foods, but high levels are found in asparagus, onions, leeks, garlic, chicory and bananas. Dandelion greens are one of the highest sources of fructans, as are Jerusalem artichokes, or products made from them. Barley, rye and wheat are also good sources, although wheat comes with its own set of other drawbacks as discussed earlier. Fructans act similarly to fiber, but do not actually create bulk themselves; instead they promote bulk by encouraging the growth of healthy bacteria in the colon — as much as popular probiotics such as acidophilus cultures in supplements and yogurt. In many people, prebiotics can actually help healthy colonic bacteria replace unhealthy bacteria that commonly cause disease.

While improved colon health can help prevent constipation, diarrhea and other functional problems, it can also help prevent intestinal diseases including cancer, and serious inflammatory conditions such as ulcerative colitis and Crohn's disease. Other bodywide benefits may include prevention of heart disease, other cancers and even osteoporosis. In addition, fructans help the colon produce certain nutrients, including biotin, vitamin K and some of the B vitamins. As opposed to some fibers, such as wheat fiber, which can prevent calcium, iron and other minerals from being absorbed, fructans can actually improve mineral absorption. This is the reason for a positive relationship between fructan intake and prevention of osteoporosis.

Cooking can reduce the availability of prebiotics in a food by 25 to 30 percent, so try to eat enough of the raw vegetables noted above. Loss of fructans occurs in cooking water, so when cooking these foods be sure to consume the water too.

Fructan supplements have appeared on the market over the last few years, as both inulin and oligosaccharides. The natural version of inulin is extracted from chicory root using only hot water, filtration and drying. Unfortunately, most versions are highly processed and have been synthesized from sugar. Synthesized fructans are also used in the manufacture of fake food ingredients — both for artificial fats and low-carbohydrate foods. For most people, obtaining sufficient fructans can be accomplished by eating more foods containing them.

How Much Do You Need?

So how much fiber and prebiotics should you eat? By now you should know the answer to this question — it depends on your individual needs. On average, between 15 and 25 grams of fiber per day is the absolute minimum most people require. This works out to be about 10 grams per 1,000 calories. Many people need more fiber than this, and some people may need twice this much, or even more, to have optimal health. As you determine your carbohydrate needs, balance your fats and start eating 10 or more servings of vegetables and fruits per day, you should notice whether your intestines are working better, or if you need more fiber and/or prebiotics.

Prebiotics should not be counted as part of the fiber requirement — instead, they should be consumed in addition to fiber. The symbiotic relationship of prebiotics and fiber mean that consuming proper amounts of these substances will improve the functionality of both. While there are no specific recommendations for the amount of prebiotics you should consume, Americans eat on average only about 1 to 3 grams of fructans daily, while our healthier European friends consume three times that amount. This does not necessarily mean that more is better, but most people will benefit by eating more food fructans.

If you don't get enough fiber naturally from foods in your daily diet, you may need a dietary supplement. The best way to do this is to make your own mix of fibers. This may require some experimentation, but it will be worth the effort. For many people, plain psyllium is all that's needed. Others, for example, may try a mixture of psyllium and oat bran, mixed with applesauce (a good source of pectin). A quick analysis of your diet should give you an idea of how much fiber you're getting, and how much more you'll need.

Both fiber and prebiotic foods are very important aspects of health and human performance. As you go through this book making changes in your own diet you'll most likely have little trouble determining whether you need more fiber and prebiotic foods based on the function of your intestines.

16

Water, Water, Everywhere

The three macronutrients — carbohydrate, protein and fat — are often the key focus in discussions on nutrition. In this book, we've expanded on those to discuss vegetables and fiber as other very important dietary components. But there's another nutritional component that's at least as important as these others. This nutrient is water. Pure, clean water can be the most essential of all nutrients. You can live for weeks without consuming food, but go more than a few days without water and your very survival will be at risk. Proper intake of water is so vital to optimal function that a deficiency of less than 1 percent can begin producing signs and symptoms of dysfunction. Slightly more dehydration can produce serious health problems. The key to maintaining proper hydration is to drink plenty of water throughout the day.

Water is the key ingredient in maintaining chemical balance in your body. This includes transporting nutrients to the cells, maintaining the function of blood, and eliminating wastes from the lungs, skin and colon. Water also plays a major role in hormone regulation and balancing acid-base levels. More importantly, water is like your car's radiator, cooling the reactions that create heat in your body. For example, muscle contraction, digestion and the processing of nutrients produce large amounts of heat, which must be cooled by water. If this regulation did not occur effectively, your temperature would rise to a level that would destroy your enzymes and other protein-based substances, and you would die. The water literally absorbs the excess heat and carries it to the skin, where it is dissipated through evaporation and other means.

About 60 percent of the body is made up of water, with different areas accounting for various percentages. For example, about 80 percent of your blood, heart, lungs and kidneys is water; your muscles, brain, intestines and spleen are about 75 percent. Even areas like your bones, which are 22 percent water, and fat stores, 10 percent water, require a specific level, which, if not maintained, results in poor function.

One of the biggest problems of dehydration is that it decreases blood volume. Maintaining blood volume is important because so many vital functions are associated with it:

- Transport of oxygen-carrying red blood cells to muscles.

- Transport of nutrients, including glucose, fats and amino acids.

- Removal of carbon dioxide and other waste products.

- Transport of hormones that help regulate muscular activity.

- Neutralization of lactic acid to maintain proper pH.

- Maintenance of efficient cardiovascular function.

Most of the body's water is contained inside the cells of muscles, nerves, organs and even the bones. This water helps regulate the intracellular environment. Water also functions in between the cells by helping to carry nutrients and hormones into the cells. One of the most significant functions of water is to regulate the balance of potassium (on the inside of the cell) and sodium (outside the cell). This balance is most important in nerve and muscle cells, producing nervous-system function and muscle contraction.

Preventing Dehydration

Thirst is how most people remember to drink water. But this is a problem, since the brain's thirst center does not send a message until you are almost 2 percent dehydrated. By then, you already have problems associated with dehydration. The kidneys, however, respond to dehydration much sooner than the brain tells you you're thirsty, another good example of your body giving you signals. In this case, if your urine output is diminished, you're beginning to dehydrate. What is meant by diminished? If you're not urinating at least six to eight times each day, you may be dehydrated. But the color of your urine may be the best and earliest indicator that you need more water. Urine should be clear, except for the first urine in the morning because you're mildly dehydrated then and drinking water should be one of the first things you do upon awakening. If your urine has a yellow color, it probably means you need more water. The darker the yellow the more water you need.

Water input must balance water loss, which occurs from several areas of the body. Most water is lost through the kidneys. This water is used to help eliminate waste products from the body. But during vigorous activity, such as exercise, the body attempts to conserve water, and loss through the kidneys is very limited. Evaporation from the skin, important for controlling body temperature, is also a major source of water loss. Even under cool, resting conditions, about 30 percent of water loss occurs here. But sweating, from exercise or normal daily activity, increases this amount dramatically — during exercise, it's about 300 times the amount lost during rest! Water loss in exhaled air is also significant. The air going in and out of your lungs needs to be humidified. And a small but significant water loss (about 5 percent) occurs through the intestine.

The amount of water loss is determined in part by air temperature (the higher the temperature the more water loss), humidity (drier climates result in more water loss) and body size (the larger the person the more water loss). If you're dehydrated, just drinking a glass of water won't solve the problem. Complete water replacement throughout the body may take 24 to 48 hours no matter how much you drink at one time. Unfortunately, the human body does not function like that of many other animals. By drinking a large volume of water, dehydrated animals can consume 10 percent of their total body weight in a few minutes, and rehydrate. Humans need to drink water in smaller amounts much more frequently to correct dehydration and maintain proper hydration.

What should you do to prevent dehydration and maintain proper hydration? Here are some general everyday guidelines:

- Don't wait until you're thirsty to drink water. Drink water every day, throughout the day.

- Drink smaller amounts every couple hours rather than two or three large doses a day.

- Have a water bottle near you at all times, and get into the habit of drinking water. Especially keep water near your immediate area during work hours or where you spend much of your time (at your desk, by the phone, in your car).

- Avoid carbonated water as your main source; the carbonation may cause intestinal distress.

- Get used to drinking water before and immediately after exercise. If you exercise for more than about an hour, drink small amounts of water during the workout.

- Learn to drink water without swallowing air — drink slowly and without tilting your head up and back.

- Remember that the average person may need about three quarts of water each day.

- Avoid chlorinated and fluoridated water.

In addition to the above recommendations, get used to drinking water as your main source of liquid. While it's true you obtain some of your water needs through food and other beverages, most should come from plain water, consumed between meals. Certain drinks such as coffee, tea and alcohol can actually increase your need for water because of their diuretic effect (causing the body to lose water). So don't count these beverages as part of your water intake. (Even decaf coffee and tea can contain small amounts of caffeine.)

Is Your Water Safe?

Only 1 percent of the world's water is safe to drink. Today, more people are questioning not only the quality of their drinking water, but the container it comes in. If you are concerned about your health, you should not just assume your water is safe to drink — you need to take active steps to find out for sure. And if there is a problem you need to correct it. Most contaminants in water fall into four categories:

- Environmental chemicals, including pesticides, herbicides and trihalomethanes, a by-product of chlorination, and chemicals that can leach out of plastic bottles.

- Heavy metals including lead, copper, and nitrates.

- Bacteria, including the most common coliform bacteria.

- Radiological pollution, including radon, radium and uranium.

If you're concerned about your water, the first step is to analyze it to find out what, if any, contamination exists. Once any questions about the quality of the water are answered, necessary steps to improve it can be taken more logically. The first question to ask is in regard to the source of your water. For most people, this is either a public water system or a well.

Individuals on public systems have the legal right to ask for and obtain the results of past water tests from their water supplier. The supplier must also inform you of any problems, past or present, in meeting federal requirements for safety. The supplier can also tell you if your water contains chlorine or fluoride.

If your source of water comes from a well, you'll have to take the initiative and have the water tested yourself. If you've recently purchased your home, a water test should have been done before the sale. At other times, the health department may do certain tests, especially if there are local pollution problems. Deeper wells generally have less contamination than more shallow, often older, wells. Even if your area has a safe environment, many problems can come from water runoffs and chemical leaks far away from your well.

Whether you drink public or well water, another potential source of contamination is your pipes. The biggest problem is potentially found in older houses. Because lead is a serious health hazard, lead pipes and lead-containing materials were outlawed in 1986. However, in older houses (built before 1930), the plumbing may include lead pipes, lead-containing solder or other lead-based materials. These soft, dull-gray metal pipes are very dangerous, especially with soft water. Some cities, like Chicago and New York, may have lead connector pipes, which connect the city water supply to homes. The water department or city engineer should be able to tell you whether this is the case with your home.

Copper pipes can also leach copper into your drinking water. High copper levels occur in areas where there is soft water (sometimes referred to as a low pH or high acidity). Although not as serious as lead, excess copper can cause health problems, including disturbances of mineral balance, especially zinc, iron and manganese, with excess copper being stored in the liver and brain.

Some homes, especially in the northwestern United States, have older pipes or tanks made of galvanized steel. This metal can leach cadmium, and, as with copper, this may pose health dangers.

Corrosion of pipes can also cause excess contamination. This is typical in areas where basements are damp year-round. The most common source of corrosion is from the grounding of a home's electrical system. This is easy to inspect. Electrical ground wires should never be attached to your water pipes, but to a separate ground.

Although the most accurate method of analyzing your water is through a lab, observing the stains in your sink may be a clue to some contaminants. The exception is lead, which won't render any discoloration. Copper, however, will produce a blue-green stain, and iron a brown streak.

Having your water tested by a competent laboratory will remove all the guesswork regarding its safety. Samples should be taken from a frequently used source, such as the kitchen sink. A morning sample would generally have the highest levels of mineral contamination, as water sitting in the pipes all night tends to accumulate these substances. For this reason, let your water run a few seconds or more in the morning or whenever water has stayed in the pipe more than six hours, to allow that water to be discarded. If water sources in your area have been contaminated, or if several members of your household have symptoms which may relate to contaminated water (such as recurring diarrhea or vomiting) the health department may do testing. The health department may also give you names of reputable labs that can test your water. These labs use Environmental Protection Agency (EPA) standards, and although some feel the EPA's ranges of normal are too conservative, at least you are ensured accurate testing.

The lab may want to provide you with special collection containers, as some samples need to be properly preserved.

In some instances, such as in the case of high lead content, you may ask your doctor about testing the levels in your blood. The EPA has changed the standard for this toxic metal from 50 parts per billion (ppb) to 10 ppb when testing home water. But even at low levels, a long-term buildup in the body is always a possibility. Children are most susceptible to lead toxicity.

If you still have questions about your water, the EPA has a "Drinking Water Hotline" in Washington, D.C.: 800-426-4791. It can provide you with a list of contaminants and the allowable levels. If you find contaminants in your water supply, there are several things you can do to remedy the problem. If the source can be corrected, such as your septic or lead pipes, this becomes an obvious priority. If the source cannot be found, a water-filtering system can usually solve your problem.

Fluoride Safety

The issue of fluoride and its safety is lengthy and complex, and I won't attempt to cover the debate here. But I do want to address the use of fluoride as an additive to drinking water. I'm basically opposed to having fluoride in the water supply because it is a high-dose synthetic supplement used out of its natural environment. And, we're all forced to consume it, whether we need it or not. Instead of treating everyone with fluoridated water, an attempt should be made to target those who really need it. In the case of cavity prevention, it would be better to treat susceptible individuals than to treat entire water supplies.

More effective than fluoride in the prevention of tooth decay is maintaining proper oral pH. Some foods, mainly carbohydrates, are acid-forming. Many commercial toothpastes also make the mouth more acidic. An acidic environment in the mouth promotes tooth decay. Conversely, a more alkaline environment prevents decay. Certain foods, such as cheese, some toothpastes, and baking soda, as well as natural fats and oils will leave the mouth more alkaline. Honey is one carbohydrate food that can also make the mouth more alkaline, and also help reduce dextran, a sticky substance that enables bacteria to stick to the teeth. Oral pH is especially important before bedtime. For children, a glass of apple juice or milk just before bed can promote tooth decay, and fluoride won't necessarily remedy that problem.

Despite what most people think, fluoride is no longer considered an essential nutrient. Natural fluoride is found in most foods, especially chicken, fish, seafood and tea, and it's found naturally in most drinking water. Through a healthy diet, enough fluoride can be consumed to have a positive effect on cavity prevention. The National Institutes of Health (NIH) says tooth decay has declined sharply in recent years, even in areas without fluoridated water. British researchers also found, after studying people from eight different countries, that tooth decay was declining equally in both fluoridated and non-fluoridated areas.

Fluoride can also negatively affect other areas of the body — especially the bones. Some studies show that fluoride can substantially increase bone loss, producing bone fractures in the spine, wrist and arm. Other studies have shown that in communities that have fluoridated water, hip fractures are more common.

Fluoride also interferes with energy production. This occurs in the anaerobic biochemical pathways that convert sugar to energy.

About half the water systems in the U.S. have fluoridated water. If you wish to avoid fluoride, either use bottled water or filter what comes through the tap. However, some bottled water contains fluoride (ask the company or read labels), and most water filters don't remove fluoride. The best filter for this purpose is a reverse-osmosis system.

Filter Your Water

The first step in considering a water filter is learning what contaminants are in the water. Once you know what needs to be filtered, you can use the appropriate system. Unfortunately, there is no single water filter that will solve all your potential water problems. Keep in mind that toxins also can enter the body through the skin or lungs when taking a shower. For example, the inhalation of trihalomethanes, a cancer-causing chemical, during showering in chlorinated water is a common problem. This can be remedied by using a system that filters all water entering your house, or by installing a water filter on your showerhead.

The three best water filters include activated-carbon systems, reverse-osmosis systems and distillation units. Each one will filter specific contaminants.

Carbon filters, dating back to the ancient Greeks and Romans, trap contaminants as the water passes through the filter. Solid-carbon-block filters are the most effective for this process (as opposed to granular-carbon devices). Carbon filters remove most organic chemicals, such as pesticides and herbicides, chlorine, bacteria, metals (lead, iron, copper) and radon, but they do not remove all minerals (so they won't soften water), or other compounds like arsenic, nitrates, viruses and radioactive particles. Carbon filtration usually improves the taste of the water. Some carbon filters contain silver nitrate to prevent bacterial build-up; these filters may have the potential to leak silver, which is toxic. Ideally, the carbon cartridge must be replaced periodically to maintain effectiveness and normal water flow. Small carbon-filter units for water bottles are also available, making safer water possible when you are away from home.

Reverse osmosis has been used for large-scale projects, such as industrial desalination of seawater. Essentially, it's a more complex filtration system that includes carbon. Reverse osmosis removes toxic metals and radiation contamination, except radon, but does not remove many organic chemicals.

Distillation, like carbon filtration, is also an ancient method of treating water. This is the best all-around method, as it "filters" more items than any other single device, although it is not technically a filter process (it's more like rain water, made from evaporating water that becomes clouds). The process involves boiling the water to be treated, and capturing and cooling the steam, which gives you cleaner water. Distillation removes toxic metals and radiation contamination, except radon, and also removes minerals and thus softens the water. It may not remove all organic chemicals.

Manufacturers of these different filtering devices can provide you with more information on which contaminants they remove as well as proper use, installation and maintenance costs. Also, it's well worth testing your water again after installing a water filter to be certain it is performing properly.

Water (and other foods) stored in plastic containers may not be as safe to drink as once thought. For many years, plastic has been suspect regarding the possibility that harmful chemicals contained in many plastic materials can leach into water. As research continues showing this is a real hazard, there are a variety of things we can do. Here are some recommendations:

- Avoid using plastic as long-term storage containers for water or other foods. Instead, save all your glass containers to use for food storage.

- Certain foods react strongly with plastic. Avoid buying vinegar, tomato, alcohol and similar products contained in plastic.

- Remove the plastic parts to bottles containing these foods. For example, some bottles of vinegar contain plastic pouring spouts which can be removed.

- Use glass bottles for water when away from home.

Drinking adequate amounts of clean water is another key to building optimal health and human performance.

17
Dietary Supplements

Throughout this book I have emphasized the need to eat real food and avoid processed, synthetic and artificial products. The same holds true when it comes to dietary supplements. However, the most important focus on nutrients should be the diet, not supplements. Always try to obtain all your nutrients from healthy, real-food. When there is a need for supplements, because of an increased nutritional need or the inability to obtain certain nutrients in adequate amounts from a healthy diet, supplementing with products made from real foods is the next most effective approach.

There are several distinctions you need to make before deciding to supplement your diet. The first is whether you actually need a supplement. This can be accomplished in a variety of ways. The first is with the help of a health-care professional who may determine this through a variety of ways; from a good history, blood and urine tests and other evaluations. However, with some exceptions, blood and urine tests generally are not the best ways to determine nutritional needs — although they can uncover serious deficiencies. Other ways to determine your potential needs for supplementation include experimentation, diet analysis, and symptom surveys. These options are discussed below.

Some people may effectively determine the need for a dietary supplement through careful experimentation. Even a doctor, who may determine the need for a particular nutrient, is experimenting by giving or recommending a certain nutrient. Whether from a health-care professional or done by yourself, the best determination that you need a particular nutrient is that it makes something better; this may include the successful treatment of a particular problem or the elimination of an abnormal finding in a blood test or other evaluation. In almost all cases, this should not take much time. For example, if you have asthma symptoms and want to see if the nutrient choline is needed by your body to help improve your asthma, taking choline for a month or two will almost always either help, or do nothing. If it helps, you may want to continue taking choline but also find the foods high in choline so your diet may provide more of it (in this case the best food source is egg yolks).

Another way to determine the need for a dietary supplement is to analyze your diet. This is a common tool used by health-care professionals, researchers and even individuals to evaluate nutrient intakes. This makes use of a computerized program and provides your level of nutrients compared to the recommended daily allowance (RDA) or other standard reference (such as the USDA's Dietary Reference Intakes or DRIs). Large national surveys are also taken the same way, and these continue to show seriously low intakes of many nutrients. For example, a Department of Agriculture survey showed that 80 percent of American women did not achieve RDA levels of folic acid, iron, zinc, vitamin B-6, magnesium and calcium.

I used various computerized diet analysis programs during my years in practice, and tested almost all patients. Just as other surveys have shown, most people had serious nutritional imbalances. Today there are many computerized diet analysis programs available, and the USDA website (www.usda.gov) provides a simple online program that is free.

If specific nutrients are found to be below a minimum level, then first you are in need of dietary improvement to include or increase foods containing these nutrients. Second, you may need additional nutrients from a dietary supplement.

Another approach that can help determine the potential need for a dietary supplement, and one used throughout this book, is the use of health surveys. This approach is based not on nutrient levels in the body or in food but on how your body uses its nutrients. These surveys utilize certain signs and symptoms associated with too much or too little of specific nutrients. They may offer clues that point to a specific nutrient, or a condition that may be associated with a nutrient. For example, sleepiness after meals, a larger waist size and frequent hunger and craving for sweets may indicate an excess intake of carbohydrates, a macronutrient. Fatigue, excess blood loss and the habit of chewing on ice may indicate the need for iron, a micronutrient.

Unfortunately, many people are led to believe they need a dietary supplement through other unreliable means — advertising, newspaper and magazine articles, a next-door neighbor ("it works for me!").

If you determine that you do need to supplement for a particular nutrient, there are several things to consider. The fact that a dietary supplement contains nutrients does not mean it's natural, or even safe. The vitamins in most dietary supplements, for example, are synthetic. And, research is showing that many forms of dietary supplements are dangerous.

Beware of HSAIDS

First, most dietary supplements on the market do not provide vitamins and minerals as they naturally occur in real food. Although these supplements may be labeled "natural," their vitamins are typically synthetic. And, they often provide doses much higher than foods in nature, isolated from other key parts of the food complex in which they would occur naturally. Specifically, these high-dose, synthetic and isolated supplements usually don't contain important associated phytonutrients found in real foods. I call these supplements HSAIDS, which stands for "High-Dose Synthetic and Isolated Dietary Supplements." When consumed, HSAIDS act more like drugs than like food, thus the first major difference between HSAIDS and truly natural nutrients from foods.

HSAIDS are not necessarily bad, although some can be deadly, but they're not what most people think they are — equivalent to the same nutrient counterpart in food. The most important nutrients are those contained in foods, and if you supplement, products made from food are the best and safest choice. In some instances, such as with the careful direction of a health-care practitioner who has expertise in nutrition, HSAIDS may be required. In this case, it may be for a relatively short period of time to correct a specific condition, such as anemia. Others may have long term needs or require a very high dose of a particular nutrient, such as folic acid, to address a genetic problem. While these issues are not that uncommon, they are the exceptions. Most people do not need HSAIDS.

The primary difference between HSAIDS and products made from real food, which contain truly natural nutrients in food doses, is how the body responds to them when consumed.

Biological vs. Pharmacological Effects of Supplements

When you take a dietary supplement, there are particular physiological responses by the body. In general, nutrients in their natural state and natural dose have a biological effect, and HSAIDS have a pharmacological effect in the body.

Examples of dietary supplements that clearly act in more of a biological fashion include products made from foods, including vegetable and fruit concentrates, fish oil and brewer's yeast. These supplements provide nutrients in a concentrated form, acting essentially the same as when you consume the real food. They provide natural doses of vitamins, minerals and/or phytonutrients helping to generate energy, regulate immunity, control aging and perform billions of other functions that improve health and human performance.

Nutrients with pharmacological effects generally include HSAIDS and have actions like those of drugs rather than foods. Dietary supplements that have pharmacological effects include such common items as synthetic vitamin C (ascorbic acid), isolated high-dose vitamin E (alpha-tocopherol) and popular iron supplements. These are almost always in doses much higher than a person could possibly consume during a meal or even a day's worth of food intake — even when consuming foods naturally high in these nutrients. Many contain doses that would take weeks of eating foods rich in these nutrients to get to the same levels — in other words, five, 10, even 100 times normal amounts. By looking at the labels of supplements in a store or catalog, you will see that most, even those labeled "natural," contain doses much higher than you would get from real food and significantly higher than the RDA.

Dietary supplements that promote pharmacological activity, like most drugs, are capable of modifying body function, often in powerful ways, and are also accompanied by the risk of adverse side effects. The actions of dietary supplements with pharmacological effects can vary with individuals, and many actions are not clearly known. HSAIDS with pharmacological actions can also interfere with other nutrients, whether from the diet or from other supplements. They can also interfere with over-the-counter or prescription drugs.

As an example of the difference between HSAIDS and truly natural nutrients, consider vitamins C and E. Dietary sources of naturally occurring vitamin C, for example, have biological effects, acting as antioxidants and protecting DNA from oxygen damage. The dose in the best of meals may be 100 mg of vitamin C or less. However, the synthetic counterpart (ascorbic acid), found in almost all dietary supplements, may function differently. High doses of synthetic vitamin C, typically 500 to 1,000 mg tablets for example, can perform as an antioxidant, but can also transform to a deadly pro-oxidant — which can cause excess free-radical activity and inflammation.

Another illustration of the difference between HSAIDS and truly natural nutrients is found in vitamin E. A natural dose of vitamin E is really quite small. For example, the amount of naturally occurring alpha-tocopherol in a loaf of whole-wheat bread — a relatively high source of natural vitamin E — may be only 2 to 4 IU. In contrast, vitamin E supplements typically come in extremely high doses of 400 to 800 IU. You'd have to eat 200 loaves to reach these supplement doses. This unnatural dose of vitamin E can interfere with other more effective antioxidants and is discussed later in this chapter. And worse, these doses of vitamin E have been shown to significantly increase mortality!

Vitamins C is often sold under the "natural" label as are many other synthetic vitamins. In nature these vitamins occur with other chemical components and with associated phytonutrients as discussed later in this chapter. These supplements don't have the same function as nutrients that contain all complementary components as they occur in real food. In addition, synthetic supplements have lower bioavailability. Synthetic vitamin C, for example, is not as biologically available, and the body gets rid of it more quickly, in comparison to vitamin C in real foods. Studies have shown that vitamin C from food was 35 percent better absorbed, and excreted more slowly, than synthetic vitamin C.

There are also many potential side effects associated with HSAIDS. Consider the following:

- A cell's sensitive DNA, vital for normal function, can be damaged by consuming as little as 500 mg of synthetic vitamin C (ascorbic acid), which may be an early trigger for cancer development.

- Doses as low as 200 mg of synthetic vitamin C can act as a pro-oxidant, causing oxidative stress.

- Popular doses of vitamin C supplements can be toxic when they react with the iron in the body or iron in dietary supplements. This is because of the powerful free radicals produced by iron.

- Consuming popular doses of iron can result in excess ferritin (the body's storage form of iron), which has been associated with an increased risk of heart disease and liver stress. High iron intake can also produce damaging excess free radicals.

- Common preparations of copper, zinc or selenium supplements can be toxic and can even cause disease.

- Popular doses of vitamin K and B6 can be toxic.

- Consuming popular high doses of vitamin A can result in bone loss and may increase the risk of hip fracture in the elderly.

- Many popular HSAIDS can adversely interact with over-the-counter and prescription medications.

- In smokers, supplementation with alpha-tocopherol has been shown to increase the incidence of lung cancer.

- Consuming popular doses of beta-carotene has been shown to increase lung cancer.

- Consuming popular doses of vitamin E could increase the risk of death.

In addition to the possible side effects, there's another potential problem with taking dietary supplements — a false sense of security against the illnesses and diseases they are purported to prevent and treat. While researchers have found for decades that consumption of fruits and vegetables significantly decrease the risk of many diseases, most studies have concluded that dietary supplements containing the same vitamins and minerals do not.

Natural vs. Synthetic

Consumers of dietary supplements are often confused as to what is a truly "natural" product and what is not. Many synthetic vitamins are erroneously referred to as "natural" because their chemical structures are sometimes identical or similar to the real thing. Even if you don't take a daily vitamin pill, you're probably eating some synthetic vitamins. They are added to breads, cereals and almost all packaged foods that are "fortified," as mandated by federal law since 1939. Another good reason to avoid processed and packaged foods.

As noted above, high-dose, synthetic dietary supplements occasionally may be useful, and under certain circumstances I have recommended these to patients for many years. These products can be useful in specific health conditions, serve as a stepping stone while you improve your diet to include the nutrients you're lacking, and can treat certain genetic conditions.

Isolated vs. the Whole-Food Complex

Another problem with most dietary supplements, even those made from natural nutrients, is that they have been isolated from their whole-food complexes. Not only is this quite unnatural, but in many cases the nutrients left behind are more potent therapeutically than the one that is isolated. A common example is alpha-tocopherol, also called vitamin E. Alpha-tocopherol does not normally exist alone in nature but occurs with three other tocopherols — beta, delta and gamma — and four tocotrienols — alpha, beta, delta and gamma. Together these seven other components of the vitamin E "complex" can be more important than alpha-tocopherol alone. For example, gamma-tocopherol is commonly found in natural foods and is more effective than alpha-tocopherol as an antioxidant. The common use of alpha-tocopherol supplements can be a problem since popular doses of alpha-tocopherol can displace gamma-tocopherol in the body, lowering the overall oxidative protection of the vitamin E complex.

In addition, tocotrienols are powerful substances that have potent anti-cancer actions, reduce cholesterol and perform other vital tasks. Too much alpha-tocopherol can interfere with some of these functions. For example, even moderate amounts, such as 100 IU of alpha-tocopherol, can block the ability of tocotrienols to control cholesterol.

Unbalanced, isolated high doses of alpha-tocopherol can interfere with body chemistry in other ways too. They can have a negative effect on anti-inflammatory chemical production, cause generalized muscle weakness, lower thyroid hormone levels and slightly increase fasting triglyceride levels. Like high-dose vitamin C, alpha-tocopherol may also become a pro-oxidant — which would be counterproductive to its antioxidant function.

Phytonutrients

There are thousands of nutritional components in natural foods that may even be more important than the micronutrients themselves. Many studies show that a variety of foods can protect us from cancer, heart disease and other degenerative conditions. While some assume that specific nutrients such as vitamins are responsible, it is now clear that other substances may be much more important.

These phytonutrients or phytochemicals are made by plants from sunlight (via photosynthesis) when grown in good-quality soil. These substances have been known in clinical research for decades and by practitioners of old for centuries. Scientists now know there are thousands of these natural chemicals that have potent therapeutic actions. Some examples of these nutrients are listed in the following table.

Phytonutrients comprise three main groups of plant compounds that include phenols, terpenes and nitrogen-containing alkaloids. Some of the names are familiar. I mentioned seven of them above that are part of the vitamin E complex. Other common phytonutrients include a group of carotenes (including alpha and beta, and lycopene), a group of bioflavanoids (including hesperetin and lutein), isothiocyanates that includes sulforaphan and many others. Don't be concerned about remembering all the names, but do remember to consume a variety of foods — such as vegetables, fruits, nuts and unhulled seeds such as flax and sesame — that contain the best sources of all the phytonutrients.

Some plant compounds in this category that are commonly synthesized as drugs include caffeine, nicotine, morphine and cocaine. These compounds are not considered nutrients, so the term "phytochemical" would best apply.

Some Examples of Phytonutrients

Carotenoids
- alpha- and beta-carotene
- lutein
- lycopene
- zeaxanthin

Limonene

Tocopherols
- beta, delta, gamma

Tocotrienols
- alpha, beta, delta, gamma

Isoflavones

Lignans
- sesamin

Tannins

Anthocyanins

Flavonoids
- lutein
- hesperetin
- diadzein
- naringin
- tangeretin

Isothiocyanates
- sulforaphan
- indol-3-carbinol
- crambene

Cyano-glycosides
- cocaine
- nicotine
- morphine
- caffeine

One reason studies continue to show that eating fruits and vegetables prevents cancer and most other chronic diseases, while the common dietary supplements don't, is the presence of phytonutrients. Likewise, dietary supplements made from these same foods also contain the naturally occurring phytonutrients.

More than 15 years ago, epidemiologist John Potter of the University of Minnesota, was quoted in the April 25, 1994, issue of *Newsweek*, providing us with a snapshot of the bigger scientific picture: "At almost every one of the steps along the pathway leading to cancer, there are one or more compounds in vegetables or fruit that will slow up or reverse the process." Unfortunately, most people don't eat enough of the foods that contain these powerful nutrients.

This information is not new to many in the natural health field. Going back more than 100 years, a key part of the organic movement included the theory that natural was better than synthetic and artificial. The true natural approach is to keep yourself healthy by eating real food that supplies the full spectrum of nutrients — from micronutrients to phytonutrients. Unfortunately, if you're trying to get your micronutrients from supplements, they're most likely HSAIDS — like the majority of vitamin and mineral preparations on the market. By taking these you not only risk side effects and may not be getting the whole vitamin complex, but you're missing out on the phytonutrients that accompany the natural versions.

18

Real 'Real-Food' Dietary Supplements

While many are familiar with the term "designer drugs," the same marketing hype exists in the dietary supplement industry. This is true in part because the biggest players — those that manufacture the synthetic vitamins and raw materials used to make HSAIDS — are the pharmaceutical companies themselves. The natural foods companies that make real food dietary supplements are generally very small and not yet as welcomed into the natural foods market. However, the image that dietary supplements are "natural" is prevalent, as is the marketing of supplements as "real food." But most of these claims are untrue when you read the fine print or know how products are made.

Because of the image of "natural foods," some supplements may contain food concentrates such as blueberry, broccoli, spinach, etc. However, these plant materials are not only added in minuscule amounts, they also are made from foods cooked at very high temperatures. The reason for their inclusion, as market researchers tell us, is that it looks good on the label; advertising can even include "contains real food," or some other claim about being made from fruits and vegetables. But a careful look at the label shows that the vitamins in these products, for example, are synthetic, being added separately and not from the foods. Discerning and uncovering these hidden tricks is often not easy, and many consumers are taken advantage of for a long time before learning the truth about certain products.

Another technique — I call it a trick — commonly used in the supplement industry is the use of yeast that's been fed synthetic vitamins. The technique is simple: feed a nutrient to living yeast, then dry the yeast and add it to a dietary supplement as a source of nutrients. In the case of minerals, it may be a useful technique, and claims of "natural" can be honestly made since all minerals — from calcium and magnesium to manganese and zinc — exist on earth in a natural form (most came from the sun during the earth's creation). But feeding a synthetic vitamin made by a drug company to yeast, adding the yeast to a supplement and then calling it "natural" and "real-food" is misleading to me.

Now that you better understand the difference between HSAIDS and truly natural dietary supplements, let's look at some different types of products and how they might be useful for improving health. These are some of the types of supplements I have found useful for my patients, my children and grandchildren, and that I take myself. These products include those made from whole foods, many certified organic, that have been concentrated without heat, through freeze-drying in the case of vegetables and fruits, and distillation in the case of fish and other oils. They contain therapeutic food ingredients like that of a meal or a day's worth of food. In addition to containing the specific nutrients, such as in a vitamin C product, they also contain the associated vitamins, minerals and phytonutrients normally found in the foods as they occur in nature.

Most companies don't produce supplements made from whole foods. It's difficult and costly to find foods dried with a low-heat process that preserves heat-sensitive nutrients, including the phytonutrients. It's even more difficult to find supplements made from certified-organic materials. In addition to these issues, many dietary supplements contain unwanted added ingredients. These fillers, binders and other chemicals are very common; avoid products containing casein, gluten, soy, wheat, artificial colorings, artificial flavorings and sugar.

Vitamin C Complex

As discussed above, vitamin C in nature is accompanied by many nutrients, perhaps thousands if we include the important phytonutrients that also affect fitness and health. Vitamin C is found in relatively high concentrations in certain foods, including acerola berries, citrus peel and vegetables such as broccoli. Supplements made from real food obtain all their vitamin C from these foods, as compared to synthetically manufactured vitamin C called ascorbic acid (or other versions of synthetic vitamin C).

Vitamin E Complex

Vitamin E is also called alpha-tocopherol. However, as discussed in the previous chapter, alpha-tocopherol is only one of eight compounds in the vitamin E "complex." The alpha-tocopherol fraction of the E complex does not normally exist alone in nature but usually occurs with three other tocopherols — beta, delta and gamma — and four tocotrienols that include alpha, beta, delta and gamma.

Almost all vitamin E supplements come in this isolated form of alpha-tocopherol, or sometimes in a synthetic version. Some products are labeled "mixed tocopherols" which usually is mostly alpha with very little of the other tocopherols and no tocotrienols.

Immune System

Immune-system support is the most important role of antioxidants and other immune-related compounds. Nutrients that help support the immune system provide maximum protection against the onset of cancer and other chronic disease. As discussed later in this book, one important purpose of certain immune nutrients is to help the body produce its most powerful antioxidant called glutathione. In addition to natural forms of vitamin C and E, other nutrients that promote glutathione antioxidant activity include lipoic acid, the amino acid cysteine (sometimes in the form of N-acetyl-cysteine) and sulforaphan, a sulfur compound in cruciferous vegetables such as broccoli, kale, Brussels sprouts and cabbage.

Two- to three-day-old broccoli sprouts (before their leaves turn green) have the highest levels of sulforaphan. Traditional antioxidant supplements are void of these naturally occurring powerful compounds. Both alpha-tocotrienol and gamma-tocopherol are also more powerful antioxidants than either alpha-tocopherol or vitamin C.

Other phytonutrients, including limonene, naringin and tangeretin support the process of apoptosis — a reaction that triggers the death of cancer cells. These compounds are found in the skins of citrus fruits. An ideal supplement to support immune function may also contain key elements in real foods such as the full spectrum of carotenoids, including lycopene, along with health-promoting compounds found in turmeric and ginger.

Whole-Food Multiple Supplements

The natural counterpart to the synthetic multiple vitamins is the whole-food multiple-vitamin/mineral supplement made from real foods. Ingredients for these products include a variety of vegetables such as kale, Brussels sprouts, beets, carrots, broccoli, spinach and parsley; fruits such as citrus and berries; and natural brewer's yeast, which contains B vitamins. These supplements contain a food dose of vitamins, minerals and phytonutrients, and, since they're made from real food, they probably contain nutrients not yet discovered!

Omega-3 Fats

Omega-3 fat from fish oil is one of the best nutrients to improve fat balance. In my practice, I found through dietary analysis that significant numbers of patients were deficient in omega-3 fat. It has been estimated that more than 50 million people in the United States are affected by essential-fatty-acid imbalance. Omega-3 oils are most useful in reducing the condition of chronic inflammation. Fish oil contains both EPA and DHA, vital for many aspects of optimal health and fitness, especially combating inflammation. A variety of other foods complement this task, including ginger, garlic, turmeric, citrus peel and sesame oil. When buying oil-based dietary supplements, read the labels: make sure the oil has been tested for oxidation and for heavy metals and other potential toxins found in the oceans. A good guide is to use fish oil labeled as containing "0" cholesterol. Many have levels of only 2 or 4 mg of cholesterol, but this may infer they may not have been cleaned of potential toxins.

Some people take flaxseed oil as an omega-3 supplement. However, there are two important factors to mention again. Since flaxseed oil is extremely susceptible to oxidation when exposed to air or heat, it is best to purchase it in capsules. And, flax oil does not contain EPA. Conversion to EPA in the body is not very effective, and requires vitamins C, B6, niacin, and the minerals magnesium and zinc.

Black-Currant-Seed Oil

Black currant seed yields a high-quality omega-6 oil containing gamma-linolenic acid (GLA) which is converted to the group 1 anti-inflammatory eicosanoids. People with allergies, especially in the spring when natural series 1 eicosanoid levels are low, often need this supplement. GLA is also essential for carrying calcium to muscle and bone cells. Without it, the calcium in your diet won't be as useful and some may be stored as calcium deposits. Borage oil and evening primrose oil also contain GLA. It's important when taking any product containing GLA to also take EPA (fish oil) or raw sesame-seed oil. These oils help prevent GLA from ultimately converting to arachidonic acid, which promotes inflammation. Both sesame and all the GLA-containing oils are also very sensitive to oxygen, and should be purchased in capsule form.

Vitamin B Complex

Along with vitamin C, the B vitamins are the most common synthetic vitamins in the marketplace. Almost all B vitamins in health and drug stores, whether the whole B complex or single vitamin products, are synthetic. In the case of the B vitamins, those that are synthetic are also referred to as inactive — in order for the body to utilize these vitamins they must be converted to an active form, which takes other nutrients and energy, and is not always effective.

As is the case with natural vs. synthetic vitamin C, the body may not utilize the synthetic B vitamins as well. In fact, up to 30 percent of the population may be unable to utilize synthetic folic acid.

Below is a list of some truly natural/active forms of B vitamins:

- Thiamine (B1): thiamine pyrophosphate and thiamine triphosphate

- Riboflavin (B2): riboflavin-5-phosphate

- Niacin (B3): nicotinamide adenine dinucleotide (NADH)

- Pantothenic acid (B5): pantethine

- Pyridoxine (B6): pyridoxal-5-phosphate

- Folic acid: 5-methyl tetrahydrofolate and folinic acid

- Cobalamin (B12): methylcobalamin

The B vitamins are important for so many functions throughout the brain and body. If levels become low, virtually any body area can break down. Those who don't get enough vitamins B1 and B2 typically are low in other B vitamins too. Here are two important surveys associated with the need for more B vitamins. The first specifically related to B1 and the second, B2.

Survey 1: Check the items below that apply to you:

❏ Carbohydrate intolerance, including diabetes.

❏ Body temperature below normal.

❏ Diuretic use (typically used for patients with high blood pressure and heart problems).

❏ Regular alcohol use.

❏ Regular caffeine use (coffee, tea, cola).

❏ Regular anaerobic exercise or athletic competition.

❏ Fatigue.

❏ Regular headaches.

❏ Reduced mental productivity.

❏ Heart problems.

❏ Poor appetite.

❏ Tendency to anxiety, phobia, panic disorder.

❏ Sleep problems.

Survey 2: Check the items below that apply to you:

❏ Skin problems.

❏ Gingivitis (gum problems).

❏ Discomfort or pain on lips, tongue or in mouth (non-dental).

❏ Cataracts.

❏ Hair loss.

❏ Anxiety, tension or personality changes.

❏ Sleep less than six to seven hours per night.

❑ Use of antacids.

❑ Pregnant (current or recent).

❑ Over age 50.

❑ Increased need for antioxidants (reduced immune function).

❑ Frequently short of breath or low hemoglobin.

The more items that apply to you, the more your levels of B1 or B2 may be too low.

High doses of the B vitamins are not well absorbed or utilized. So if a supplement is needed, it's best to take lower doses two or three times daily than one larger dose. For B1 and B2, doses above 5 mg are considered high.

Foods high in B vitamins vary considerably and are not difficult to obtain in a healthy diet. Good sources include eggs and meats; nuts and seeds, legumes, whole grains and some vegetables such as broccoli, spinach and mushrooms have moderate amounts. Significant losses occur in cooking and freezing, so raw vegetables are important sources. However, avoid the following foods in their raw state: red chicory, Brussels sprouts, red cabbage, clams, oysters, squid and other mollusks — these all contain thiaminase which destroys thiamine. Some antibiotics can also destroy thiamine. Light (especially the sun) can destroy B2, and sunlight on the skin can reduce some of the body's folic acid.

Folic Acid Folly?

Two of the many naturally occurring forms of folic acid include folinic acid and 5-methyl tetrahydrofolate (5-MTHF), the most common forms found in the foods we eat. Unfortunately, the most common form of folic acid in our food supply is synthetic folic acid. Because it is much cheaper, it is used in food fortification and virtually all dietary supplements on store shelves. This synthetic form of folic acid is inactive and must first be converted to an active form to be useful in the body.

A significant number of people are unable to absorb or otherwise utilize synthetic folic acid. The numbers are difficult to determine, but scientists have estimated that perhaps up to 30 percent of the population has this inability (which is genetically determined). These individuals must rely on natural folic acid from food, or the 5-methyl or folinic acid versions in supplements.

Natural folic acid is not just for prevention of neural tube defects, one of many types of birth defects in pregnant women. It's a necessary nutrient with bodywide benefits for all adults and children. These include the following:

- Brain function — the natural forms of folic acid are the only ones that can get into the brain. It is especially important for those who don't sleep well or are depressed.

- Intestinal function to help food digestion and absorption, heal the intestines and, as studies have shown, in preventing colon cancer.

- Important in the detoxification of substances like estrogens in both men and women to remove their harmful metabolites (this is the mechanism of breast cancer prevention as it pertains to folate).

- For protein metabolism and for regulation of certain amino acids.

- For the formation of new blood cells, which is a continuous process.

- For cardiovascular health by reducing homocysteine.

- Unlike synthetic inactive folic acid, natural folic acid does not mask anemia if not taken with adequate vitamin B12.

Calcium

Few people in industrialized societies have true calcium deficiencies, regardless of what the advertisements tell us. The bigger problem is that most people are unable to utilize the calcium they already have in their bodies. Poor calcium metabolism, rather than deficiency, is almost at epidemic proportions. The end result is that not enough calcium gets into the cells, including the bones, muscles and other tissues, with the remaining excess calcium depositing in the joints, tendons, ligaments or even the kidneys as stones. Plaque that clogs the arteries can also contain calcium.

In order for your body to properly metabolize calcium, and more effectively absorb calcium from food, you must have sufficient vitamin D. This nutrient is free and plentiful, yet most people don't have enough. That's because it comes from the sun and the public is told that the sun is dangerous. This issue is so important that it's discussed separately in the following chapter. Just remember that without sufficient vitamin D, calcium cannot be properly regulated, and that most problems of insufficient calcium are really due to low levels of vitamin D.

Another important issue regarding calcium is to consume enough calcium-rich foods; this is easily done without supplementation through good dietary practices. And it does not necessarily mean eating a lot of dairy foods. Consider the high amounts of calcium in the following single servings of non-dairy foods:

- Salmon: 225 mg

- Sardines: 115 mg

- Almonds: 100 mg

- Seaweed: 140 mg

- Rainbow trout: 100 mg

- Spinach: 135 mg

- Green beans: 100 mg

- Collards: 125 mg

Two other important issues regarding calcium are absorption (the most important part is also having sufficient vitamin D), and getting the calcium into the bones and muscles once it's absorbed.

Absorption is the first step to utilizing calcium in the body. In general, smaller amounts are better absorbed than larger amounts, whether from food or supplements. If a small amount of calcium is present in the intestine, 70 percent may be absorbed, for example, while a larger amount of calcium may have only a 30 percent absorption rate. If you're taking calcium supplements, it may be best to take a lower dose several times a day rather than a large dose once daily. Even though vegetables contain smaller amounts of calcium, larger percentages are absorbed compared to milk. So in some situations, a serving of broccoli may result in more calcium getting into the body than a serving of milk.

The stomach's natural hydrochloric acid is also very important in making calcium more absorbable. Neutralizing stomach acid has a negative effect on calcium absorption, and a serious impact on digestion and absorption of all nutrients. Once absorbed, calcium is utilized best when the body is in a slightly acidic state. Otherwise, calcium that is absorbed may be more easily deposited in joints, muscles or arteries rather than inside the cells where it's needed. The cells that are calcium-starved cause symptoms such as muscle tightness and irritability, identical to those of calcium deficiency. Morning stiffness, which loosens up only after moving around for a while, is one of the most common symptoms of this calcium problem. Signs of an advanced problem include so-called bone spurs (a deposit of calcium in the ligament) or kidney stones. Rather than needing more calcium, these people need more acidity (and vitamin D) to utilize the calcium. Two teaspoons daily of apple-cider vinegar may help maintain the proper pH to help calcium work properly. This can be taken as part of your salad dressing, or even mixed into a 4-ounce glass of water.

Excess phosphorus intake can be very detrimental for calcium utilization, pulling it out of bones and muscles. Most soft drinks contain large amounts of phosphorus — and the people who drink them risk significant calcium loss from their teeth and bones.

The type of calcium supplement may be associated with absorbability. For example, calcium carbonate is more poorly absorbed than calcium lactate or calcium citrate. This is due to the alkaline nature of carbonate, and the acid nature of lactate and citrate.

Taking too much calcium in supplement form can disturb the body's complex chemical makeup. For example, too much calcium can reduce magnesium. Most people may be in need of more magnesium than calcium — it's necessary for most enzymes to work, including the ones important for fat metabolism. And the best sources of magnesium are vegetables.

A Note on Osteoporosis

Osteoporosis is usually a multifactorial problem, meaning there's hardly ever just one cause. We know that a lack of calcium is usually not the cause, nor is low estrogen. Methods that are effective in treating or preventing osteoporosis in one person may have very different results in someone else. In addition, osteoporosis may not be as much of a problem as it has been made into, as Susan Brown, Ph.D., author of "Better Bones, Better Body" emphasizes:

- Osteoporosis itself doesn't cause bone fractures; half of those with osteoporosis never get fractures.

- Severely osteoporotic vertebrae are strong enough to withstand five times the normal weight-bearing.

- Menopause does not, per se, cause osteoporosis, and only 15 percent of a woman's bones are affected by estrogen.

- Zinc and magnesium may be as important as calcium for bones.

- Up to 80 percent of all hip-fracture patients may have a vitamin D deficiency.

Iron

Most people think of anemia when the mineral iron is discussed. But iron is an important nutrient for all areas of the body, especially the brain and the aerobic muscles; it aids in the production of neurotransmitters and other brain chemicals, is in the protective covering of nerves and helps carry oxygen in the blood to all parts of the body. Most people can obtain sufficient iron from a healthy diet, especially from beef and other meats. If supplements are necessary, because a blood test shows low levels for example, a relatively low daily dose, such as 10 mg, for a month or two may be enough. Higher doses of iron can be irritating to the intestine and very unhealthy for the whole body as discussed below. If you have a continuous need for iron, something more important may be missing.

Iron is efficiently recycled in the body, with some loss occurring through sweating during exercise, or for women, through menstruation. Excess iron loss or decreased intake may produce a serious deficiency.

Excess iron in the body can be the result of taking iron found in various dietary supplements. Iron can be deposited in the liver, resulting in cirrhosis of the liver. Excess iron is also associated with certain neurological problems including Alzheimer's and Parkinson's disease, and multiple sclerosis. Since the early 1980s, scientists have known of important relationships between high levels of stored iron and heart disease. Excess iron, even moderate amounts, may even prove to be a more significant risk factor for heart disease than excess cholesterol.

When the body has enough iron for normal use, the remainder is stored in the form of ferritin. Evidence shows that ferritin may promote the formation of free radicals. These may injure cells lining the arteries and damage heart muscle, as well as increase the level of LDL, the so-called bad cholesterol.

The marketing of iron to treat fatigue ("iron-poor, tired blood") may be one reason for excess accumulation of iron in some people, as iron supplements are still very popular. Almost all multiple-vitamin/mineral preparations contain too much of it, and many foods are fortified with iron. Certainly, if you are iron deficient, taking an iron supplement is necessary. But without knowing whether it's needed, traditional iron supplementation should be avoided. If a blood test for ferritin shows you have too much stored iron, the first thing to do is assess whether you are consuming too much. Often, excess iron stores are the result of an accumulation of iron over several years. The use of iron cookware also can contribute to high iron stores. In some situations, the body's metabolism may not be functioning properly, resulting in excess ferritin. Donating blood may be one way to help reduce excess iron stores.

A Note on Choline

Like all essential nutrients, choline is required for most of the body's basic functions, but one out of 10 Americans don't get enough. Choline is critical for proper fat metabolism, preventing the deposit of fat in the liver, transporting of other nutrients throughout the body, and is associated with the adrenal glands' regulation of stress. Choline is also very important for the brain in the production of acetylcholine, and in particular with memory. Egg yolks and fish are excellent sources of choline in the diet. A common indication for the need for choline supplementation is asthma. Wheezing, coughing from bronchial spasm, and excessive mucous production during exercise has been termed "exercise-induced asthma" (although it occurs more in those who don't exercise) and is typically associated with a need for choline. Normally, the body's response to activity or exercise is to dilate the airway passages to allow for better air passage. In exercise-induced asthma, this dilation is followed by excessive narrowing of the air passages. Choline can help the nervous system control proper bronchial action. In this situation, a high dose of choline may be needed initially; for example, 500 mg several times daily until breathing improves.

Case History
Roy was a slim, 44-year-old construction worker who wanted to "run with the guys" after work, though he could run with them for only about 15 minutes due to his severe asthmatic reactions. This was due in part to the stress of running at too high a heart rate without proper training, but also a need for choline. After two weeks of taking choline, his symptoms were gone. Eighteen months later, after improving his aerobic system and eating eggs daily to keep his choline intake adequate, Roy qualified for and competed in the world masters' track and field meet in Australia, where he won a box full of medals.

Skin and Hair Care
The best nutrition for healthy skin and hair starts with a great diet, especially balanced fats, adequate protein, good intestinal function and proper hydration. Adequate circulation of blood, discussed later, is also very important. If your skin or hair is very dry and unhealthy, or you have other skin problems, this is usually a sign of reduced health, including the need to improve the diet. Focus on total health, not just skin and hair. While this topic could fill a whole book, this

book is about getting and staying healthy, which would include skin and hair.

Here are some specific recommendations for skin and hair care:

- For sun protection, a number of nutritional substances can be effective. These are nutrients you can take internally rather than topically as a sunscreen. Your body uses up a number of substances rapidly after sun exposure. These include folic acid, beta-carotene and lycopene. Tocotrienols, from nuts and seeds, and a part of the vitamin E complex, can help protect the skin directly, and limonene, found in citrus peel, can protect against skin cancer. All the antioxidants also help with sun exposure since increased free radicals are one harmful effect of too much sun. In addition, fish oil, by mouth, helps protect the skin during sun exposure.

- Many skin problems are associated with low or deficient levels of vitamin B2.

- Pure shea butter is a unique skin-care product made from an African nut extract (similar to a coconut) and has been used for centuries as a beauty product. European studies have shown that shea butter is remarkably active against skin blemishes and irritation. It's also useful as a daily hand, face or body ointment. As a moisturizer, it is helpful against the damaging effects of the sun and also helps maintain the skin's elasticity.

- Pure coconut oil is also great for the skin.

- The omega-6 fat GLA is perhaps the best remedy for localized skin problems. Breaking open a gel cap of black-currant-seed oil and rubbing it into the skin is a great remedy for dry skin, wrinkles, or even the most stubborn skin problems, as good if not better than other expensive skin remedies on the market. It's also good for burns, including sunburn, but only after the skin has been thoroughly cooled.

- Finally, don't put anything on your skin you're not willing to eat! That's because you absorb most ointments, creams, lotions, soaps and other items commonly used on the skin and scalp. Most especially avoid fragrance, which is listed on the label as such. Use only plain, pure liquid and solid soaps without chemicals — not an easy task when shopping but these products are available. Some are scented with lemon, peppermint and other natural oils.

The most important factor associated with dietary supplements is not any particular supplement, but that you should try obtaining all your nutrients from a healthy diet. Only after you've done the best job with your food intake should a dietary supplement be considered.

19

Let the Sun Shine!

We should love the sun because we can't be healthy without it. Humans have been in sunny environments since the beginning. The sun offers a free source of vitamin D, and is the primary source of this important nutrient that has powerful effects in the body. Vitamin D allows us to more effectively use calcium, improves the immune system and helps prevents cancer and other diseases.

Not until the past few decades has the incidence of skin cancer become such a problem. This period also corresponds with the development of sunscreen and other products that attempt to block the sun's rays. William Grant, Ph.D., who has published many papers on this issue, says that sunscreen is overrated and gives a false sense of security. Other research shows the use of sunscreen can actually increase the risk of malignant melanoma (the most common and deadly form) and other skin cancers. Grant and other researchers describe the problem this way: Most sunscreens block ultraviolet B waves (UVB) very effectively, but do not block longer-wave more dangerous UVA well. We obtain vitamin D through UVB, and if we block that wave sun-stimulated vitamin D production is reduced.

The false sense of security that sunscreen gives many people causes some to stay in the sun longer, exposing the skin to more dangerous UVA, and increasing risk of skin cancer. For this and other reasons, the growing list of research supports the notion that we can prevent a significant number of many types of cancers by spending some time in the sun, without sunscreen. This includes the prevention of skin cancer.

Some studies show a relationship between sunscreen use and cancer prevention while others have not. Unfortunately, sunscreen manufacturers and cosmetic companies spend millions on marketing, using popular scare tactics to convince people to use their products.

Based on recent scientific studies, currently recommended vitamin D levels are inadequate, even with the recent increase in recommendations. The average daily need for vitamin D is about 4,000 IUs, but the current recommendation is still only in the 400 IU range from birth to age 50. Recent studies show that more than half the population has inadequate levels of vitamin D — and some of these studies were done in the sunny states of Florida and Arizona!

In addition to calcium regulation and prevention of cancer, vitamin D specifically helps reduce pain caused by various types of muscle and bone problems. The sun also plays an important role in immunity, especially in children. And, the sun is good for the brain — getting natural sunlight helps the brain work better. No, not staring into the sun, but allowing the eyes to be exposed to natural outdoor light (contact lenses, eyeglasses, sunglasses and windows block the helpful sun rays).

Children and the Sun

Coralee Thompson, M.D., says "many children, especially those with brain problems, are deprived of vitamin D and some are outright deficient, which severely affects brain function." Disabled children, for example, also have a very high incidence of osteoporosis due to calcium wasting secondary to low vitamin D levels. (The same scenario can occur in anyone at any age.) A common problem that's not often discussed is the fact that bone loss later in life is significantly related to a lack of sun exposure and vitamin D levels during childhood. And, most of the damage that causes skin cancer in adults occurs during childhood.

"Kids need to be in the sun without sunscreen for short periods of time based on individual needs," says Dr. Thompson. "This may be 15 minutes building to 30 minutes a day for the average skin type, but never allow a child to get sunburned." Most clothing allows some sun to get through for vitamin D production. Dr. Thompson cautions that, "dietary supplements of vitamin D are not as effective because the oral dose is usually too low, and higher levels of vitamin D are potentially toxic." Interestingly, high amounts of vitamin D obtained from the sun are not toxic.

Stay Tan

For most of my career I have recommended getting a good tan to protect the skin against excess sun damage. In fact, tanning provides protection similar to sunscreen, and with protection specifically against the potentially dangerous UVA. A recent issue of *Science* (March 2, 2007) says the same: "A dark natural tan offers unparalleled protection against skin cancer." Not everyone can tan. Very fair-skinned people, those with red hair and those with freckles, can burn quite easily, and these individuals must be very cautious.

Following are three important factors to consider when it comes to the sun:

- **Use the Sun Wisely.** Everyone knows that spending the afternoon lying on the beach in the strong summer sun is not healthy (although people continue doing it). But we need sun exposure. Children need sun too, from an early age. But like adults, they should never stay in the sun long enough to burn. If you work in the midday summer sun you should cover yourself — a hat and light, long sleeves are usually sufficient, but some people may need more protection. Those who are sun-sensitive should avoid midday sun, and sometimes even late morning and mid-afternoon summer sun. Most people who are sun-sensitive already know it. In this case it's important to take a natural vitamin D supplement as food sources of this nutrient are inadequate.

- **Eat Right.** The very best skin care products are nutrients found in the healthy foods we eat. Essential fats, antioxidants, vitamin A and other dietary nutrients offer the greatest skin care *and* the best protection from natural sun. Vegetables and fruits provide most of these nutrients, with fish oil, egg yolks and whey products offering other valuable factors.

- **Don't Eat Sunscreen!** Again, my recommendation has always been to not put anything on your skin you're not willing to eat! That's because sunscreen, along with so many things people put on their skin, gets absorbed into the body. A tan can protect skin from sun overexposure, as can a hat and light clothing, and avoiding midday sun during summer months.

The sun is our primary source of vitamin D, and the only way to get it is by spending some quality time outdoors. Vitamin D not only helps us utilize calcium better but helps prevent disease, including skin cancer and many internal cancers.

20

Eat, Drink and Be Merry

Now that I've covered many issues about foods, this chapter discusses how to further implement this understanding into your daily life. Topics such as snacks, shopping, cooking and food preparation and other eating and drinking issues are in this chapter. Healthy food should be tasty, easy to buy and prepare, and most importantly, every meal and snack should be a joyous occasion! While many people take great pride in the car, entertainment center or front lawn, it's most important to take pride in your health.

Food should not only be healthy, but festive — among the top pleasures in life is a delicious, satisfying and healthy meal. Too many people have lost their natural inclination for this sensation. We should eat, drink and be merry if we want to live long and healthy lives. That does not mean we should abuse food and drink. Instead we should know what and how much to eat and drink, and our merriness should be genuine. At one time, people instinctively knew what to eat. Today, large corporations spend billions of dollars telling us what we're hungry for. And it works. But the responsibility you have is to your body — making it healthy and maintaining it for a long and wonderful life

Snacking Your Way to Health

Thus far we've discussed what to eat, and how to balance it, but there's yet another component to healthy eating habits that can make a positive difference in your health — how often you eat. Specifically, eating more frequently, or snacking between major meals, can improve your health in many ways. In fact, perhaps no other single dietary habit can make a more positive difference in your health than healthy snacking.

In our society, snacks are generally seen as an unhealthful addition of unwanted calories and fat, and something to avoid. This can be quite true if you snack on junk food such as candy bars, snack cakes, chips and crackers that are full of sugar, refined carbohydrates and unhealthy fats. But healthy, real-food snacks have many health benefits and can help provide you with a continuous supply of the fuel necessary for optimal human performance. Research clearly shows that healthy snacking can help you control blood-sugar levels, improve metabolism, reduce stress and cholesterol, burn more body fat and increase energy levels.

A healthy snack is just a small meal. And, the key to healthful snacking is to reduce the amount of food eaten at regular meals, and distribute this nutritional wealth throughout the day. Eat five or six smaller meals that add up to the same amount of food that you would normally consume in a typical two- or three-meal-a-day routine. The ideal plan is to start the day with a good balanced breakfast that includes an adequate serving of quality protein. For example, a vegetable egg omelet, a bowl of plain yogurt and fruit or a healthy smoothie can get your day off to a good start. Skipping breakfast may be one of the worst nutritional bad habits, but worse yet is eating a high-carbohydrate breakfast of cereal or a bagel, which can be counterproductive, negating all the effects of this more healthy style of eating. From breakfast on, plan to eat every two to four hours, based on how good it makes you feel. Those under more stress or with blood sugar problems usually need to eat more frequently — especially initially, when eating every two hours can quickly make significant changes in overall health.

An example of a daily meal schedule starts with breakfast, a mid-morning snack, lunch, a mid-afternoon snack, a light dinner, and if necessary a small snack (which can be a healthy dessert) later in the evening.

Healthy snacks can be almost anything you like, just as long as they are made from real, healthy food. For many people, snacks, like regular meals, should contain protein. Experiment to discover how much food you need and which types work best. Some people may need to eat much larger snacks but others can get by on minimal amounts like just a small handful of raw almonds. Snacks should be just like any other healthy meal, just smaller, and still supplying adequate nutrition. This might include:

- Vegetables and fruits such as an apple or pieces of carrot and celery.

- Raw almonds or cashews, or combine almond butter with apple slices.

- Leftovers are always easy snacks.

- Plain yogurt and fresh fruit.

- Cheese and fruit.

- A boiled egg.

- Homemade energy bar or healthy smoothie as discussed later.

The benefits of healthy snacking are many. They quickly suppress cravings, especially for junk foods, they improve physical and mental energy, and can even stimulate fat-burning by changing your metabolism. Since snacking stabilizes blood sugar and prompts your body to produce less insulin, your body will store less fat and use more of it to fuel all your daily activities from work to play. Many people find that they have much more energy when following a program of healthy snacking.

Snacking can also help your body counteract the harmful effects of daily stress. In this way you reduce the over-production of the stress hormone cortisol, as well as insulin. Both prompt your body to store more fat.

Snacking also helps to reduce cholesterol. Studies show that eating more frequently can lower blood cholesterol, specifically LDL, the "bad" cholesterol. In addition, studies show a staggering 30 percent increase in heart disease in those eating three meals or less per day.

While snacking has received a bad rap over the years, experts now agree that it was the type of food, not the frequency of eating, that caused problems. In addition, just piling on the calories by adding snacks to an already unhealthy diet is clearly dangerous. Now we know that eating healthy, balanced snacks throughout the day can help you improve your health in many ways.

A favorite snack food is my homemade Phil's Bar. Use it as an in-between meal snack, as a meal when traveling, and even as a healthy dessert. It's a complete meal, low glycemic, high in protein and contains good fats. The recipe follows:

Phil's Bars
3 cups whole raw almonds
2/3 cup powdered egg white
4 tablespoons pure powdered cocoa
1/2 cup unsweetened shredded coconut
Pinch of sea salt
1/3 cup honey
1/3 cup hot water
1 to 2 tablespoons vanilla

Grind dry ingredients. Mix honey, hot water and vanilla. Blend into dry ingredients (at this point, you may have to mix it all by hand if your mixer isn't real efficient). Shape into bars, cookies or lightly press into a buttered muffin tin. You can also press the batter into a dish (about one inch deep) and cut into squares. Sometimes these are better when allowed to dry. Adjust the water/honey ratio for less or more sweetness. Keep refrigerated (they'll still last a week or more out of the refrigerator). For other flavor options, use fresh lemon instead of cocoa, or use more coconut.

Need a fast snack — right now? Grab an apple. Or make a "bar in a cup" — a tablespoon of almond butter in a cup with some honey. Healthy options are endless, so create your own list.

Tips for Healthy Cooking

How and if you cook your food can be just as important as how you select it, since even the healthiest ingredients can be reduced in quality through improper kitchen practices. The biggest problems are overcooking, using too-high heat, and overheating certain types of oils. Following are some guidelines that can help make your work in the kitchen become a work of health.

The worst method for cooking anything is deep-fat or high-heat frying, especially using vegetable oils. While many healthy foods may be lightly sautéed in butter or olive oil, deep-frying overheats the oil and can be deadly. In addition, the high heat may destroy other nutrients in the food itself. Meats, fish and poultry can be grilled, roasted or cooked in their own juices with sea salt. Less oil or butter is needed for pan-cooking meats because they often contain sufficient fats. Additionally, most people overcook meats and destroy some of the valuable nutrients. It's also important to not use too-high heat for too long. For instance when grilling a steak, remember to turn it every minute or so to prevent the excess formation of chemicals that can be harmful to your health. This goes for vegetables as well — if using high heat, turn them often.

Vegetables can be steamed, stir-fried in olive oil, roasted, baked or grilled. Cook vegetables minimally to avoid destroying vitamins and phytonutrients — they also taste better when not overcooked. If boiling or steaming, use as little water as possible to avoid leaching of nutrients.

Eggs can be soft- or hard-boiled, or cooked sunny-side up, over-easy, poached or lightly scrambled. Use low heat to avoid "tough" or rubbery eggs.

If using oils for cooking it's important to remember that all oils contain varying ratios of monounsaturated, saturated and polyunsaturated fats. Monounsaturated and saturated fats are not sensitive to heat, but polyunsaturated oils are very prone to oxidizing when exposed to heat. This oxidation produces free radicals, which are related to many health problems. Butter is one of the safest oils for cooking, as it contains a low amount of polyunsaturated fat. Olive oil can also be used for cooking but its polyunsaturated content is a little higher. Another fat you may consider for cooking is coconut oil. In addition, try lard, which contrary to popular belief may be a healthier choice for cooking than butter.

Eat Raw Foods

Consuming a significant amount of fresh, raw food is very important for optimal health. You need not be obsessed with raw food, but make sure you're getting some at each meal and that the majority of foods on your menu are fresh and raw.

Rediscovering Lard

You've probably been programmed to believe that the absolute "worst" fat you can consume is lard. Well, that's a commonly held belief, but consider the facts. Many people are surprised to learn that compared to butter, lard contains more heart-healthy monounsaturated fat, and less saturated fat and cholesterol. A tablespoon of lowly lard contains 5.7 grams of monounsaturated fat compared to 3.3 for butter. Lard weighs in at 5 grams of saturated fat compared to 7.1 for butter. And lard contains less than half the cholesterol of butter — 12 mg compared to 31 mg. Lard also contains less heat-sensitive polyunsaturated fat than olive oil — 1.4 grams compared to 2.

For these reasons, lard may be a better choice for cooking than butter or olive oil. Many chefs prefer it for its flavor and its ability to withstand heat. And it's relatively inexpensive, too. However, if you decide to use lard for cooking, it's important to seek out an organic source, since toxins often accumulate in the fats of animals that are not organically raised.

Mention raw foods and most people think of a big salad. But there are so many different ways to add not only raw vegetables and fruits to your diet, but other foods as well. Here are some ideas:

- A garnish for any dish — parsley, large leaves of lettuce or cabbage under a cooked piece of meat or fish.

- A small serving of fruit between appetizer and entrée to "clear the pallet."

- Fruits or berries for dessert.

- Chopped raw nuts or seeds on top of various foods, including healthy desserts.

- Raw milk cheese and yogurt.

- Olive and coconut oils.

- Raw honey.

- Foods that are slightly cooked on the outside, but raw on the inside: rare or medium-rare beef, lamb or fish, and eggs (lightly fried, poached or soft boiled).

The nutritional quality of foods is affected by cooking, and by deep freezing and other common factors associated with food storage. Individual nutrients may be adversely affected by a number of factors that reduce their levels in food. Consider the following:

- Many nutrients are affected by cooking, including vitamins A, C, thiamine (B1), riboflavin (B2), pantothenic acid (B5), pyridoxine (B6), and E, as well as biotin, the carotenoids and folic acid.

- Glutamine, lysine and threonine are amino acids unstable to heat. The more they are heated, the more is lost.

- During cooking, significant amounts of nutrients may be lost in liquids that are not consumed.

- Compared to fresh foods, both freezing and canning can reduce nutrients. For example, niacin loss in frozen vegetables may be 25 percent and in canning 50 percent.

- Foods stored for longer periods may lose nutrients, even when they are still "fresh." After 48 hours, for example, lettuce may lose 30-40 percent of its vitamin C content.

- Ripened foods generally have higher levels of nutrients. Tomatoes have more vitamin C and beta carotene when ripe compared to unripe; bananas have more vitamin C when ripe compared to medium ripe.

- Some vitamin E is destroyed by cooking, food processing, and deep-freezing.

- Dietary supplements should also be made from raw foods. These should be labeled as such — not just vegetable and fruit concentrates, but freeze-dried concentrates, which are made through a slow, cold evaporative process. Most supplements don't use foods carefully concentrated because they cost up to 10 times the prices of foods dried with high heat. The most common process is a high-heat (400° F) process.

Kitchen Tips and Equipment

Preparing food should be enjoyable and result in delicious meals. A problem for many people is they are not familiar with real food preparation, or don't have the right tools to make the work easy. While there's nothing like experience, jump right in. Here are some helpful tips.

A well-stocked kitchen also contains various hand utensils, electric items and other gadgets to accomplish interesting things. For example, a simple spiral vegetable slicer can create long thin "spaghetti-like" pieces of raw zucchini. Top it with a beef and tomato sauce for a delicious Italian meal.

Other useful utensils include a mandolin slicer, glass bowls for mixing and storing, wooden cutting boards, high-quality knives, a garlic press, a grater (including a fine one for fresh ginger), a citrus peel slicer, and a small hand citrus juicer for use in recipes.

In addition, the two most frequently used appliances in my kitchen are a food processor (I have a Cuisinart but any good brand will work) and a very good blender (I have a Vita-Mix). If you're buying organic meat in bulk, a grinder (to make fresh ground meat) and/or a slicer is very useful.

Glass and heavy-duty stainless steel pots and pans provide the cookware. Avoid all aluminum, copper and non-stick products due to the potential for food contamination. Iron cookware is also good except avoid using high-acid foods in them, including tomato and vinegar.

Shopping for Health

An important step you can take for better dietary habits is to properly shop for the food items that will bring about the greatest health. Bad food has less of a chance of getting into your body if it never gets into your grocery cart. With proper planning, you can make sure only healthy items get into your cart and your body.

Begin planning your shopping trip before you leave home. Never shop or make a shopping list when you are hungry because you will tend to buy unhealthy items. Instead, have a snack, make a list and decide which store or stores offer you the healthiest choices. Many cities now have health-food supermarkets, and many of the larger chain groceries now carry higher-quality foods, such as organic produce. Just beware of organic junk food and other tricks of the trade.

In most grocery stores, you will find that the real-food items are usually stocked on the store's perimeter. While making this loop, try to buy as few items in packages as possible. If you do buy items in packages, always be sure to read the label and study the list of ingredients and nutritional facts. If the item contains anything that does not promote health, it belongs back on the shelf and not in your cart. In addition, choose organic items when available. Stick to your list. Remembering everything on it will keep you focused and help you avoid such dietary pitfalls as the fresh-baked French bread (full of refined white flour and fake vitamins) that grocers place strategically and aromatically at the ends of store aisles.

Your most important stop on the store perimeter is the produce section. Choose a variety of fresh greens and vegetables for salads and cooking. Avoid starchy potatoes and corn. Once again, look for organic produce, especially if you are buying spinach or celery, as these crops are often heavily sprayed and can retain high pesticide residues. Also in the produce section are fresh fruits. Minimize the high-glycemic fruits such as large bananas and watermelon, and instead choose fiber-rich apples, pears and grapefruits, and phytonutrient-rich berries.

Next stop is the meat section. Seek out natural or organic grass-fed beef, pork and lamb, free-range poultry and wild-caught ocean fish. These more-natural meats can be found in many supermarkets and health-food groceries.

Bakeries are usually located on the store perimeter — pass them by. The deli counter may have some items that are whole and healthy, but most are not; be careful.

Also on the outer edge of the grocery you will find the dairy section. If you must buy milk, consider goat milk. Cream, butter, plain yogurt and cheese are items to consider. Look for organic items, since toxins such as pesticides and hormones often bind to the fat in dairy products.

Near the dairy section are the eggs. Most stores now carry organic eggs. They cost a little more but are still an inexpensive protein bargain.

If you stick to the perimeter of the store, you'll find that you only rarely need venture up an aisle. Usually the only food items you'll need up the aisles are extra-virgin olive oil, raw unfiltered honey, beans, nuts, nut butters, spices and sea salt.

Milking Your Health

A wise old axiom is "cow's milk is for calves, human milk is for humans." Unfortunately, most people hear the "Got Milk?" ads and ignore professional recommendations. Milk consumption is up, and so are the problems created by it. In many people, milk can cause various types of gastrointestinal stress, skin problems and lowered immunity to infections and allergies. And worse is the potential for hormones and chemicals, so especially avoid milk and milk products that are not organic.

Milk allergy is common in adults and children. In most people, milk allergy symptoms are delayed and not obvious until it's eliminated from the diet. These delayed reactions come in many forms; eczema, asthma, constipation, chronic nasal congestion, gastroesophageal reflux and others. In some people, there is an immediate allergic reaction by the body's immune system, usually to the casein protein. Symptoms typically include swelling, itching, hives, abdominal cramping, breathing difficulty and diarrhea. In a severe reaction, hypotension or shock can result. Lactose, or milk sugar, poses another potential problem with milk, as many people have difficulty digesting this sugar and some cannot digest it at all. Those who have difficulty digesting lactose do not produce enough of an enzyme called lactase, which breaks down the complex lactose into simple sugars. In these people, the lactose ferments in the small intestine, producing gas, bloating, cramps and diarrhea. Lactose-digestion problems are also associated with more serious problems such as irritable bowel syndrome, premenstrual syndrome and mental depression.

Many people who have problems with cow milk find that they can tolerate milk from sheep and goats much better. Goat milk is widely available in many grocery stores and is lower in lactose. The fat in both goat and sheep milk is made up of smaller fat globules that are easier to digest. The protein structure of goat and sheep casein is also less allergenic than cow casein.

Wine, Alcohol and Your Health

Wine is not only the oldest alcoholic beverage but the oldest medicinal agent in continuous use throughout human history. The use of wine dates back more than 6,000 years, and is attributed to physicians, scientists, poets and peasants. Even today, wine and other alcoholic beverages are classified as foods and used daily in most cultures. More healthful benefits have been bestowed upon wine than any other natural substance. For instance, drinking wine with meals can help with relaxation and digestion.

There are few known unhealthy effects from moderate amounts of alcohol consumption, with negative consequences seen mostly in those who go beyond moderation. In fact, as we've all heard for a long time, there are many positive health benefits associated with wine consumption. Drinking wine and other alcohol in moderation significantly lowers the risk of coronary heart disease. Moderate drinkers have healthier cholesterol ratios as alcohol raises the HDL and lowers LDL. This may be one reason for the lower incidence of heart disease in consumers versus abstainers. Another may be that alcohol increases blood flow to the heart. In addition, alcohol reduces the tendency to form blood clots, a major cause of heart attacks (and strokes). Alcohol also lowers the risk of Alzheimer's disease and other types of dementia, and improves bone health. Moreover, those who don't drink actually have greater risk for heart disease. Some scientists say that people who have one or two drinks per day may add three to four years of life expectancy, as compared to those who don't drink.

Scientists also say that red wine may be a potent cancer inhibitor. Resveratrol, a substance found in red wine (due to the fact that grape skins are used to make red wine, but not white), grapes, and thousands of medicinal plants from South America and China, not only interferes with cancer's development, but may also cause precancerous cells to reverse to normal. Resveratrol also has anti-inflammatory properties.

Most wine contains about 12 percent alcohol (mostly ethanol, with only a very small percentage of other types of alcohol). Sweet dessert wines may contain up to 20 percent alcohol. This compares to 40 percent (80 proof) and 50 percent (100 proof) alcohol in distilled products such as vodka and gin. Wine also contains vitamins B1, B2, B6 and niacin, as well as traces of most minerals, including iron. Most red table wine contains iron in the easily usable ferrous form. The pH of wine is low, like that of the stomach; perhaps one reason wine improves appetite and digestion. Eating natural fats with wine slows the absorption of alcohol and protects the intestine from possible irritation.

Once in the blood, alcohol is broken down in the liver. About 3.5 ounces of pure alcohol can be safely metabolized by the body if spread out over the day. This translates to about a bottle of wine — not something I'm recommending. To a European, this may not seem like excess, but to an American it might. In the United States, the average annual per-capita consumption of wine is just a few teaspoons, while in Italy, it's about a half bottle.

As a group, women are more susceptible to negative effects of alcohol because of their smaller size, and because they have less amount of alcohol dehydrogenase in their stomachs and livers. This enzyme breaks down much of the alcohol before it's absorbed, and in the blood.

If you enjoy wine and want the health benefits associated with it, drink only what you enjoy and can tolerate, and no more than one or two glasses. The simplest recommendation is a 4-ounce glass or two with meals. For most people a glass of wine will be completely metabolized in about an hour and a half. Some people, however, should never consume alcohol. But a moderate amount for those who can, and want to, is now considered to be 4 to 8 ounces of wine per day.

An obvious side effect of alcohol is that it impairs your senses, so it should be avoided within four hours of driving a vehicle. One drink increases the risk of an accident by 50 percent, two drinks by 100 percent. Also, wine should not be taken with other drugs, or by people with certain illnesses, and is not recommended for pregnant women. Although wine gives a relaxed feeling, any alcohol can disturb sleep if consumed shortly before bedtime. Studies of biological circadian rhythms in humans show that alcohol is best metabolized between 5 and 6 pm. If you enjoy wine, be sure to ask your doctor whether it poses any health problems for you.

Caffeine: Coffee and Tea

Many people use caffeine as a drug, as a means of getting more "energy." If this is the case with you, you may be addicted. And if you need a drug to give you a pick-up, your fat-burning system may not be working very well. Caffeine can also induce adrenal, liver and nervous-system stress, and create unstable blood-sugar levels in many people. As with everything else, you must determine whether your body can tolerate caffeine from coffee or tea. If you can, there are some important considerations. Buy your coffee beans as freshly roasted as possible, keep enough in your cabinet in a tightly sealed glass container and the rest in the freezer. Grind them just before you make the coffee. The lighter roasts have more caffeine, and the darker roasts less. Just as with fruits and vegetables, it's best to choose organic coffee to avoid pesticides and other chemicals.

Many health benefits have been associated with both green and black tea, including anti-cancer properties, since they contain a variety of antioxidants and phytonutrients. Once again, organic tea is better than conventional as tea growers may use many pesticides.

Good News for Cocoa Lovers

The evidence is growing that cocoa is a powerful therapeutic food. Including this treat in the diet may do more than satisfy a craving — it may also help to improve health. Cocoa can help lower blood pressure and improve cardiovascular health. The flavanols found in cocoa, purple grape juice and tea can stimulate processing of nitric oxide, which promotes healthy blood flow and blood pressure, and cardiovascular health. In addition, recent research confirms other studies indicating that flavanol-rich cocoa may work much like aspirin to promote healthy blood flow by preventing blood platelets from sticking together.

Real, unsweetened cocoa typically contains significant protein, about 7 or 8 grams per ounce. It is also low in carbohydrate — between 8 and 13 grams per ounce, with 50 to 60 percent or more of that carbohydrate coming in the form of fiber. Like other beans, cocoa contains many vitamins and minerals, including folic acid, niacin, zinc and magnesium. The fats in natural cocoa also have healthy attributes. More than a third of the fat in cocoa is monounsaturated. An equal amount of fat in cocoa is in the form of stearic acid. Though saturated, stearic acid is a good fat, as it can reduce LDL cholesterol. Cocoa also contains the essential fat linoleic acid.

Cocoa also has strong antioxidant benefits, which have also been shown specifically to protect against LDL-cholesterol damage. One study showed that when a cocoa snack was substituted for a high-carbohydrate snack, it increased the "good" HDL cholesterol and reduced blood triglycerides. And, it did not increase LDL cholesterol despite being a higher-fat snack. Polyphenols in cocoa, similar to those in red wine, provide protection against blood-vessel problems, including heart disease.

While cocoa has some very healthy attributes, eating it in a candy bar is not recommended since this usually includes a lot of sugar, bad fats and chemicals. Only buy pure cocoa — without sugar or dairy — and use it to make your own healthy desserts, sweetened with honey.

Caffeine content of some single-serving drinks

(Amounts in milligrams of caffeine. Amount varies with how you make it, product and size.)

Regular coffee 85-300

Double espresso 120

Decaf coffee 3-5

Black tea 50-140

Green tea 20-50

Real cocoa 25-50

Most herb teas don't contain caffeine. But some over-the-counter drugs do in a range of 15-300 mg (read labels).

Salt of the Sea

If you use this universal ingredient, sea salt can be a flavorful and healthful addition to your food. Sea salt usually tastes better than regular salt, and contains other minerals as well. Early humans obtained much of their food from the salt-water ocean, and we still require many of the sea's vital minerals.

People have come to fear sodium these days, almost as much as fats. However, like certain fats, sodium is an essential nutrient. Sodium is necessary for water regulation, the nervous system, muscle activity, adrenal gland function and many other healthy activities. Sodium intake through a healthy diet, with the addition of added salt, is the best way to obtain sufficient amounts for most healthy people. For those who sweat a lot, or perform high levels of exercise, sodium loss increases through sweat. Those under excess stress, and athletes who are overtrained, may have hormone imbalances that can cause too much sodium loss through the urine. These individuals sometimes crave salt, and usually need to consume more.

Sodium can increase blood pressure in susceptible individuals. This occurs in about one-third to one-half of those with hypertension. In these cases, too much sodium can cause edema and/or further elevation of blood pressure. This sensitivity can be discovered through an examination by a health-care professional, and by avoiding salt and sodium for a week and checking how blood pressure changes. Most patients with high blood pressure can correct the problem when the proper amounts of carbohydrates are determined, especially beginning with the Two Week Test. This can often reduce or eliminate sodium sensitivity.

Spice Up Your Health

Spices have been used in food preparation for thousands of years. The right spice, or combinations, can make foods tempting and delicious by boosting the appearance, smell and taste. Spices also are useful as natural preservatives, and many have powerful therapeutic and health-promoting properties, too. In food, spices can prevent the growth of dangerous bacteria and other organisms. And when ingested, they can fight against cancer, heart disease and other chronic conditions. All these benefits come from the healthy oils, antioxidants and phytonutrients. Here are some examples:

- Oregano, thyme and bay leaf can protect against potentially harmful infectious agents such as Candida, E. coli, Salmonella and Staph, and even the potentially deadly Klebsiella pneumoniae.

- Turmeric contains the antioxidant curcumin and has powerful anti-inflammatory (and cancer preventive) properties, as does rosemary.

- Ginger has powerful anti-inflammatory properties, and can inhibit the rhinovirus — one of the viruses responsible for the common cold. Hot ginger tea, made from fresh ginger and a small amount of honey, is one of the best remedies when those around you are getting a cold or you feel it coming on. Ginger's antioxidant properties are at least as effective as those of vitamin C, can be very useful for nausea and motion sickness, and help protect the intestine from ulcers. In addition, ginger may have properties that promote fat-burning.

- Capsaicin, found in hot red chili peppers, also has anti-inflammatory properties, and can stimulate increased oxygen uptake, which is one reason it may also increase fat-burning capability.

- Wasabi, a hot root used with Japanese foods, also protects against potential food poisoning by bacteria and fungus. It also contains anti-cancer properties, including powerful antioxidants.

- Parsley and cilantro not only add a visual pleasure to a plate of food but are full of therapeutic phytonutrients.

- Fenugreek (the seed) contains high levels of flavanoids, which are important antioxidants, and has been shown to have cholesterol-lowering capabilities. This spice can also reduce platelet aggregation (important for proper blood flow) and reduce blood sugar in diabetics.

Many other herbs and spices have therapeutic value as well, including cinnamon, allspice, nutmeg, cloves, dill and basil. These can be found fresh in groceries or can be grown in your garden, window box or even an inside window sill. Dried spices can lose not only their flavor but also their therapeutic value over time, as many potent substances break down. And, since they contain polyunsaturated oils, they can go rancid. Buy spices in small packages, and keep them sealed tightly and stored in a cool, dark place.

Deadly Doughnuts

Love the taste of doughnuts? If you want to be healthy you better get over it. Even though some are "cholesterol-free," these crispy items are one junk food to avoid. Their bad ingredients include trans fats, sugar, refined flour, artificial flavors and colors, and many other chemicals with names you can't pronounce.

But there's more danger — the ingredients tell nothing of what really gives doughnuts their unique crispy flavor. Most doughnut makers buy oil that other fast-food operations have already used to fry their products. This tired oil often has been used to fry other foods for weeks. The intense heat breaks down the oil and turns some of it to soap. This combination gives doughnuts their special crispy taste and texture; something that fresh oil fails to do. There are many other flour products made with used oil out there as well, so beware.

The main problem is that these oils — including trans fats — adversely affect the delicate balance of fats in your body, producing too many cancer-promoting eicosanoids. Along the way, inflammation, increased blood pressure and other problems can be triggered too. Even just one doughnut contains enough of these dangerous fats to remain in the body and trigger unhealthy actions for months.

21

One Last Bite

There are always questions and other topics that just cannot be addressed in a book, and that's one reason for this new 5th edition. As new research helps confirm earlier ideas or if modifications and additions are made, these are left for another time and place. My website — www.philmaffetone.com — addresses many of these other issues including new topics. For now, I want to highlight some common topics regarding food that need mentioning, and offer more tips to get you on your way to a new you.

The concept of individuality is very important, yet people still either miss it or use it as an excuse to not eat in a healthy way. No one "diet" can work for all individuals. And clearly, this book does not offer any one diet but instead, information and ideas that you can use to help individualize your eating plan. It's really an education in intuition.

Some people say they feel better eating junk food, and so, they rationalize, that must be the best way for them to eat. Sorry, if you really believe that notion then not only is this book not for you but all that junk food adversely affected your brain. There are basic, natural rules we all must follow when it comes to eating right. For example, we must all drink adequate amounts of water for good health as one day of low intake can put stress on many areas of the body. Avoiding processed food is another natural law as even one serving of refined sugar, for example, can have a significant adverse effect on your health. Avoiding bad fats is equally important considering that a meal with hydrogenated fat, for example, can remain in the body and do damage for a couple of months. Nor do we want to be obsessed with eating; the stress created by being fanatical about minor details, for example, can outweigh some of the benefits. The answer? Balance all of the healthy things in life while avoiding the unhealthy ones — a basic foundation of this book.

Beware of advertising! It distracts us in our efforts to live healthfully. It's negative education — propaganda. These shameful activities, frequently directed at children, have completely reshaped the modern world's eating habits. In less than a century we've gone from a diet high in natural foods to one made mostly of highly processed harmful items. No one should be surprised at the prediction that in the next decade 75 percent of our population will be overfat; chronic life-threatening diseases are already affecting people at younger ages than ever before, including children.

Unfortunately, the so-called "natural foods" movement of today is not helping. Synthetic vitamins, processed and packaged convenience items, and organic junk food is now the norm, making up most of the items in health food stores.

Your job, should you choose to accept it, is to avoid all the hype. For every bad food, it seems like there's a new diet associated with it. While the low-calorie, low-fat and other diet plans don't work very well, they're still the most popular. Let's look at some of them.

Counting Calories

The calorie-counting theory is based on the idea that the calories in the food you eat minus the calories you burn for energy equals the weight you lose or gain. The idea is that balancing energy intake and output results in stable weight. If you eat fewer calories than you burn, you lose weight, or, if you take in more than you use, you gain. The problem with this theory is that it does not work as simply as it seems for most people. This is because everyone has a slightly different metabolism, food is utilized differently, and fat and sugar are burned at different ratios from person to person. For example, some people get 60 percent of energy from fat and 40 percent from sugar, while others are just the opposite. When you hear "burning calories," your question should be, "calories of what — fat or sugar?" (This issue is related to your aerobic system as discussed later.)

In addition to the number of calories taken in, the amount of carbohydrates, fats and proteins eaten also significantly affects how the body burns energy. So to use only the total calories as a guide may be misleading. More importantly, counting calories doesn't work in real life for most people, and the side effects can be significant — the least damaging being long-term weight gain as a result of slowing down your metabolism on a calorie-restricted diet.

Case History
When Sally turned 30, she decided to get serious about taking off the excess weight. So she followed a low-calorie diet that limited her intake to 1,000 calories per day. Within three months, Sally felt more tired, but finally reached her goal of losing 20 pounds. Within six months, she gained about 25 pounds back. She went back on her diet, and it was just as successful as before, although it took a little longer to lose the 25 pounds. This vicious cycle continued for about five years. Sally was now not only tired, but depressed, had insomnia, and had PMS for two weeks each month. During my initial consultation with Sally, I explained how she was continually suppressing her metabolism and getting more unhealthy with each vicious cycle. Sally was weaned off her calorie-counting and eventually was able to eat as much as her body required. In time she got down to the same size clothes she wore when she was at her "ideal" weight at 22 years of age. And to her surprise, she was eating about 2,000 calories each day!

Calorie counting almost always results in eating less food. When you eat less food, especially less fat, which contains the most calories, one of the significant results can be that your metabolism slows down and you can eventually store more fat, despite your initial (short-term) weight loss. That's why so many people eventually gain more weight and fat after being on a calorie-restricted diet. The best way to speed up metabolism is to eat the amount of good-quality food you need each day, including fats, and be physically active.

Low-Fat Diets
One of the most popular and health-damaging diet plans is the low-fat diet. The basic idea is built on the fallacy that calorie-dense dietary fat causes the most weight gain and is detrimental to health. Many people on low-fat diets have a "fat-phobia." Low-fat diets are popular among calorie-counters because they are a seemingly easy way to reduce calories.

There are several problems associated with low-fat diets, many of which are the same as those associated with low-calorie diets. Low-fat diets can slow metabolism, and also increase hunger through reduced satiety. People on low-fat diets tend to eat more carbohydrate; as you may recall, 40 percent or more of carbohydrate is directly converted to fat for storage by the body. And, many low-fat packaged foods are higher in sugar; with the fat content lowered, the flavor is gone too, and manufacturers must add sugar to make it more palatable.

The worst problems associated with low-fat diets are essential-fatty-acid imbalances, hormonal problems and disease. Essential fatty acids are usually deficient in low-fat diets, along with all the benefits previously explained. Women who are on or who have been on low-fat diets are especially vulnerable to hormonal imbalances. And finally, contrary to popular belief, low-fat diets do not prevent disease. In fact, some types of fat are associated with prevention of heart disease and cancer.

The Gram Counter

Knowing the weight in grams of each food eaten at a meal can have more practical meaning. I've used it in this book, but primarily for reference. In addition, knowing the approximate grams of macronutrients — and the ratio between carbohydrates, protein and fat — can make it easier to relate to how the body responds, metabolically, especially in relation to insulin as previously discussed. Gram counting also includes the popular 40-30-30 plan, which suggests people eat 40 percent of their calories from carbohydrates, and 30 percent each from protein and fat. Soon after starting private practice, I used this ratio as a starting point — not as a "cookbook" diet — but to help people further determine their individual needs. Calculating the percentages of macronutrients involves multiplying the grams of each macronutrient by 4 calories for carbohydrate, 4 for protein, and 9 for fat, and dividing each subtotal by the total calories of the food or meal. (Fats have 9 calories per gram, and carbohydrates and proteins each have 4 calories per gram.)

But counting grams, like counting calories, can also maintain the dieting obsession. Each time you eat something you have to think about how much it weighs or you have to look it up in a food table.

Most people eventually get tired of doing that and fall off their "diet." There's a better way: Follow what makes you feel the best. Follow your intuition. Why blindly follow some menu when you can do what every other animal on earth does — eat small amounts often, stop eating when you're satisfied, and eat what your body needs and what makes you feel the best.

Unfortunately, none of the popular diet approaches consider how you respond to your meals. Do they make you feel more hunger? Tired? Energized? Pay attention to how you feel immediately after a meal, and for the next few hours; one of the best indicators of whether that type of meal works well for your needs. As you consider this and other factors we've discussed in previous chapters, you'll be on your way to knowing what works best for you. What is really happening, is you're developing your natural intuition.

For many people a plan that makes sense is to determine the types and amounts of foods that work best for you, and then devise a schedule that divides this food up over the course of the day. Typically this means three regular meals with two or three healthy snacks. Eating right is often a matter of planning. You plan your day, often writing it down in your planner; you plan the clothes you're going to wear and you plan vacations. If you plan your meals as carefully, you'll be much healthier. Let's plan a sample day's menu, beginning with the breaking of your all-night fast, breakfast.

Breakfast

There's no better way to start your day than with a healthy breakfast. This includes real food, including some quality protein. Keeping your carbohydrates to the proper level will help optimize blood sugar, which will give you more physical and mental energy for the day's tasks ahead.

Of course, eggs are the perfect breakfast food. While they're not just for breakfast, they just could make your first meal of the day ideal, and a bit easier to prepare — whether poached, scrambled, soft-boiled, fried, hard-boiled or in an omelet, eggs are a quick meal.

I begin my day with a delicious smoothie. I soft boil a dozen eggs at a time and keep them refrigerated, so preparation for this is about five minutes. Here's my large, one-serving recipe:

2 soft cooked eggs.

1 large apple, pear, peach or the best in-season fruits.

1/2 cup blueberries or more per person.

1 teaspoon plain psyllium.

1 tablespoon raw whole sesame or flaxseeds.

8 ounces water.

Add all ingredients to a good blender and blend.

(The best blenders will do a great job on the whole fruits, core and all the seeds, and I include a raw whole carrot, raw spinach, kale or cilantro or other vegetables.)

Omelets are also quick, and can include a serving or two of vegetables. Just sauté some vegetables, drop in some eggs and cook either by scrambling or slowly cooking and flip. When you have more time to prepare breakfast, a fancy omelet with a sauce makes for a nice change. Another version of the omelet is quiche, made with vegetables, meat or fish. Avoid the crust and save time — just butter the dish before adding the quiche mixture. Make one or two ahead of time for another quick breakfast.

Don't have time for breakfast? Make time for being healthy. There are several things you can do to ensure you get this most important first meal of the day. First, do as much preparation as possible the night before. Not just breakfast prep, but things you do in the morning, like pack your briefcase, set out your clothes or pack your bags. As for meal preparation, get everything out and ready to go, except for the food itself; put water in the kettle, pan on the stove, plate, silverware, etc.

I have eggs every day, and with so many varieties of egg dishes there's no need to be bored with them. But maybe you still want more variety, so here's another healthy breakfast variation: yogurt or real ricotta cheese with fresh fruit. Or, leftovers. Whatever you choose to have for breakfast, just remember it's the most important meal of the day, so don't cheat yourself or your family out of it.

Lunch

If you eat a good breakfast, and a mid-morning snack, getting to lunch without crawling on your knees from hunger should not be a problem. And like breakfast, a healthy lunch is a matter of proper planning. If you're away from home, packing your own lunch usually makes for a more healthful midday meal. Arrange for that to be done the evening before so it's not another job you need to do in the morning. Plan ahead by cooking extra food at dinner so that you can include some for lunch. Eating more protein and less carbohydrate during lunch will keep you from getting sleepy or losing concentration after lunch.

A large salad is a great foundation of a healthy lunch. Use a variety of different vegetables, and dressing made from simple oil and vinegar to more elegant dressings made ahead of time. On different days you can add different proteins: meat, cheese, fish, eggs or combinations.

Leftovers from a balanced dinner make for a perfect lunch — perhaps a few slices of beef or a chunk of fish with steamed vegetables.

If you're going out for lunch, make sure you take enough time so you're not rushed, and be careful of restaurant food. Today, there are more healthy foods, including organic items, to make it easier, but ask about what's used in the kitchen. Don't be afraid to have eggs again as an option; they're a quick meal you can get almost anywhere.

Dinner

If you start the day with a real breakfast, have a good lunch, and eat healthy snacks, dinner should be your smallest meal. This is the ideal scenario. Too often, however, people do just the opposite. They skip breakfast, have a skimpy lunch and then pile on the food in the evening. Your dinner could include items from the refrigerator that you combine for a sampling of tasty leftovers you've accumulated over the past few days. Or, once again, eggs can be a great dinner. Or it could be just a small salad and some protein. Either way, dinner should be easy, delicious and relaxing.

Healthy Sauces for Tasty Meals

Whether it's breakfast, lunch or dinner, any meal can be made more savory and even romantic with a sauce. When you think of a sauce, the thought of preparation time first comes to mind. But some basic sauce recipes are quick, easy and store well. They can turn your seemingly simple and boring meals into culinary delights. Below are three basic sauce recipes that you can make with very little preparation time, and the results will keep well for use a second or third time. You may also find yourself feasting on just the sauce!

A Note About Recipes

I learned to cook by intuition, "throwing ingredients into the pot" rather than by following a recipe and measuring everything. I recommend you do the same. Over time, you'll make more delicious meals in less time and without the anxiety often associated with following a recipe. I do, however, highly recommend reading through cookbooks to get more ideas about combining ingredients.

Basic Butter Sauce

The most basic of sauces is also the easiest to make — a butter sauce. When you make your vegetables, put some "sweet" butter on the vegetables when they're still hot, along with some sea salt. ("Sweet" butter is made without salt — the cream used to make this butter is a higher quality and more tasty than that used for salted butter.) Even those who never liked vegetables will usually eat them with a butter sauce. Don't be afraid to use generous amounts of both ingredients, unless there's a real reason to limit these ingredients in your diet. This is the real key to a great butter sauce. If you have the time and want to get more fancy, sauté some garlic or onions, or add some other spices (tarragon works well) into the butter. The addition of olive oil is another nice option. Prep time is just 30 seconds for the basic sauce, and less than 5 minutes for the fancy butter sauce with garlic.

Basic Tomato Sauce

This is an easy, tasty and healthy all-around red sauce. Just put some chopped tomatoes in an uncovered pot, add some sea salt and let it boil for an hour or two to reduce the water content for a thick sauce. Blending the tomatoes ahead of time is a nice option. If you can't get fresh, vine-ripened tomatoes, use canned, whole, peeled organic tomatoes which are vine-ripened and packed without preservatives. The canned ones are easier and quicker to make. When cooked down to a thicker puree, tomatoes take on a unique taste all their own and even without adding anything but salt, you'll have a great-tasting sauce. If you like tomato sauce, you'll love this simple way of making it. It's a guarantee that people who taste it will ask for the recipe! You can freeze this sauce in small containers and use it when you want. Once you have the basic sauce, if time permits, you can add other ingredients, like garlic, parsley, or a sprinkle of Parmesan or Romano cheese, or even a touch of sour cream.

Basic Cheese Sauce
This is simply made from heavy cream, butter, cheese and salt. Melt about a quarter-stick of butter, add about a cup of heavy cream, and when hot, add enough cheese to make it taste delicious — about two or three tablespoons or more. Add sea salt to taste. Grated Parmesan or Romano works great, or use your favorite cheese.

Eating on the Run
The realities of life dictate that you won't always be able to eat the way that's best. When you travel, are late for work, or somehow find you can't get a good meal when you need it, you'll have to find the best alternative. There are some acceptable options. If you're away from home and are having trouble finding good food, consider going to a deli for a chef's salad, or just some sliced meats and cheeses. Or, go to a diner for some eggs with a side of vegetables. In some restaurants, prepackaged liquid eggs are used for scrambled eggs and omelets, so get them "sunny-side up."

A great alternative is to eat a healthy energy bar. Since you'll have a difficult time finding one in the store that is acceptable, always have a batch of homemade Phil's Bars on hand.

Foods for Children
One of the most common dietary questions I receive from people relates to feeding their children. The answer, in principle, is relatively simple. From baby's first foods, they eat much the same things adults

eat, sometimes in a different form. The implementation is not always so easy, mostly due to the marketing of junk foods to children. Let's start at the beginning.

From birth, mother's milk provides everything the baby needs, including water. It's not unusual for a baby to rely exclusively on breastfeeding for all its nutritional needs through 6 or 8 months of age, or longer. I've never seen a situation where the mother was physically unable to breastfeed. If you're expecting a baby and would like more information and support on breastfeeding, contact La Leche League International (www.lalacheleague.org).

The general recommendation is to wait until at least 6 to 8 months of age before introducing outside sources of food for babies (although baby-food companies want you to think differently). A baby's intestinal tract is not yet developed to process food other than mother's milk, and the immune system could have adverse reactions to foreign foods if they're introduced too early. This could lead to intestinal distress, allergies and other problems, often for a lifetime. When babies start wanting to experiment with food after 6 to 8 months of age, you can begin trying different foods individually. If you combine more than one food at a time in the beginning and the baby has an adverse reaction, you may not know which food is the culprit. And, it's best to give the baby a choice, letting him or her choose from a variety of healthy options.

Babies are born as instinctive and intuitive geniuses; they know just what they need to be healthy. And when they start eating foods, they can self-select very well, when not influenced by adults or other kids. Studies by Dr. Clara Davis in the 1920s and '30s showed that once children are weaned, they will naturally select the foods their bodies need the most. In Davis' studies, the children developed very different dietary patterns. In the end, the children were psychologically and physically healthier than average.

Practically speaking, most parents are not willing to prepare a smorgasbord for the baby every time he or she wants to eat. But there are some patterns I discuss below that can be followed — mainly that certain foods, like carbohydrates and dairy products, should be postponed until they are more easily tolerated, and more-often selected foods should be eaten first. And, always use organic foods.

The best first foods to introduce are vegetables. Letting the baby play with a fresh raw carrot, zucchini or other raw vegetable (except potatoes since even a small amount of hidden sprout can be toxic) can be a great way to introduce food. Use larger vegetables, or pieces, so the baby can't get it stuck in the mouth. Regardless, you'll want to keep close — infants seem to get any size item into their mouths one way or another. Eventually they'll figure out they can get pieces of the vegetables with their new teeth. Try one vegetable at a time and see which they like, which, if any, they react badly to, and if they really have an interest. Some babies just want to play with food, just as with everything else around them. If they don't seem ready to eat, don't push it. Wait a couple of weeks and introduce some raw vegetables again.

Next move on to cooked vegetables — peas, squash, carrots or whatever you're eating. Just mash up the vegetables you cook for yourself and feed them to the baby. Hold the butter and salt until a couple of months later. Also keep away from rough or hard-to-digest vegetables like those in the cabbage family, including broccoli, cauliflower and Brussels sprouts. You'll gradually see what your baby likes and dislike, especially when you change diapers.

Once a variety of vegetables are tolerated, start next with fruits. Try a large piece of apple, pear or peach. Don't forget, the baby's goal is to get it into his or her mouth — whole, of course. Move on to homemade applesauce, and try pear and peach sauce too. Avoid using fruit juice; it's too concentrated, and even if you dilute it you'll increase acidity in the baby's mouth that can have a devastating effect on the teeth, leading to tooth decay later.

Now that the baby is eating fresh vegetables and fruits, you're ready to experiment with cooked eggs. Initially, try the yolk and white separately in case there's a reaction to either. Next, organic meats. Buy everything as fresh as possible, avoiding processed meats and canned foods. Make dairy and grains the very last foods you introduce. Milk and wheat are the most common allergies in children, followed by soy and corn. Why not hold off on these potential problems as long as possible since the baby will get everything he or she needs nutritionally from the other foods?

So much of the food preferences people develop later in life were acquired at an early age from what their parents fed them as babies. Starting off right makes feeding your older, potentially more picky children much easier. The bottom line is this: If your kids are not eating right it's usually your fault. In their early years, take the responsibility to buy and prepare all the food they eat. Don't let the processed-food companies and the lure of convenience dictate how your child will eat for the rest of his or her life. The quality of your child's entire life depends on it.

22

Developing Maximum
Aerobic Function

Earlier in this book I defined fitness as a crucial element to human performance. In the purest sense, fitness is the ability to perform physical activity. For most of their existence humans were extremely active, expending vast amounts of energy just to accomplish the basic tasks that kept them alive, like walking for miles in search of food. These early people had tremendous endurance based on aerobic systems that were built by their daily tasks of living. Suddenly, in just a short span of a few generations, today's humans have become much less active and as a consequence we are much more prone to dysfunction and disease. For the relative few who are physically active it's in the form of exercise, leaving the majority in a state of aerobic deficiency. But most of those who do exercise get too much of the anaerobic type, which can be very stressful, causing injury and illness.

All through this book I've emphasized the importance of burning fat for energy and optimal health. This important activity takes place in the aerobic system, which uses mostly fat as fuel. A different part of us — the anaerobic system — uses mostly sugar for energy. It follows that to improve your level of fitness, enhance your ability to burn fat, obtain unlimited energy and correct most bodily imbalances, the aerobic system must be turned on. It's up to you to develop the aerobic system optimally. I refer to this as *maximum aerobic function*, or MAF.

Your muscles have two important types of cells, or fibers. These are key parts of the aerobic and anaerobic systems. In some animals, such as chickens, the aerobic and anaerobic muscle fibers are separate, with entire muscle groups composed of one or the other type. When cooked, a chicken clearly shows this distinction — dark meat is composed of aerobic muscle, while white meat is anaerobic muscle.

In humans, muscles have a mixture of both aerobic and anaerobic fibers. The aerobic muscles make up the foundation of the aerobic system. These fibers account for the majority of muscle bulk in the human body, more than 80 percent. This fact corresponds to the ability of humans to be better endurance animals than sprinters.

Aerobic muscles have two general functions: physical activity, which helps us move and support our skeleton, and metabolic function, generating energy and other tasks. Aerobic muscle fibers physically get us through the day and they're the ones we want working during physical performance; they have the ability to work well for long periods. They allow us to sit, type and walk throughout the day; they protect the spine, hips and all other joints and bones. Without good aerobic muscle function, we're more vulnerable to joint problems, bone stress and other mechanical injuries.

Aerobic muscles thrive on physical activity. Without it, we can't be as healthy. Since most people are no longer naturally active, artificial activity, otherwise known as exercise, is necessary. The intensity of your exercise is a key factor, which I'll discuss shortly. Briefly, aerobic muscles are relatively slow-action muscles, capable of enduring easy to moderate levels of activity for long periods of time. This means you should be able to endure a long day's work without getting exhausted, and still have energy to spare. They are well endowed with blood vessels, so the more these muscles are used, the more blood flows through them and the entire body. This improvement in circulation brings more oxygen to all cells, and removes waste products, which are always being produced. Conversely, the person who is very inactive may have 70 percent of his or her blood vessels closed down!

The metabolic aspects of the aerobic muscle are the other key components of the aerobic system. Within these fibers we produce long-term energy through the conversion of fat in the muscle's fat-burning engines, the mitochondria. As fat-burning improves, the body gets an unlimited supply of energy, and the fat deposits on your hips, thighs, abdomen and even in your arteries can diminish. The aerobic muscles also help antioxidants break down potentially dangerous free radicals. Taking all the antioxidants you need won't help if your aerobic system is not working efficiently. The make-up of the diet also influences aerobic function, with high-glycemic foods (refined carbohydrates and other sugars) practically turning this system off.

Rescuing Your Aerobic System

To get your aerobic system working correctly, you must diminish or avoid factors that suppress it, and increase the factors that help it. Stress has a negative impact on your aerobic system. The different types of stress and how to control them are discussed in a later chapter. For now it's important just to know that stress of any kind programs your body to burn less fat and more sugar. The more stress, the worse this problem will be.

Dietary or nutritional factors that cause excess stress can especially inhibit aerobic function. The most common of these stresses is eating too much refined carbohydrate foods and products containing sugar. Deficiencies of essential fats or other nutrients can also inhibit aerobic development. Over-exercising is another stress that can reduce aerobic function.

If the aerobic system is impaired, energy needs switch from fat-burning toward using more sugar. This results in a real deficiency in aerobic function, resulting in a variety of signs and symptoms I call the *aerobic deficiency syndrome.*

Aerobic Deficiency Syndrome — ADS

The ADS is not an epidemic so easily defined that it makes big news each day, like AIDS, cancer or heart disease, but this problem is destroying the quality of life for many millions of people. It's one of the major causes of functional illness, and a significant contributing factor to chronic diseases such as cancer, diabetes and heart disease.

ADS occurs when the aerobic system is not well developed and maintained. This becomes a major risk factor for disease. It's no different from vitamin C deficiency, or being deprived of any other necessity of life. It can cause problems in any area of the body dependent upon the aerobic system, which is most of the body. It can affect your body chemistry causing hormonal imbalance, your physical body causing hip, knee or back problems, or your brain resulting in depression. By now, you know what causes ADS. In general, the two most common causes of ADS are:

- **The underuse of aerobic muscles**. It's the simple rule of "use it or lose it." Only a small percentage of the population is naturally active — their day-to-day work activity is relatively high. And, few people perform proper aerobic exercise.

- **The overuse of anaerobic muscles**. Most exercisers overtrain not by volume but by performing too much anaerobic activity, such as weight-lifting, or activities performed at too high an intensity.

Other common causes of ADS, as noted above, include consumption of too much carbohydrate, including sugars; low-fat diets; and stress.

When asking yourself about the status of your aerobic system, do an inventory of all the functions with which the aerobic system is associated. The symptoms of ADS are many; the most common ones include:

- **Fatigue.** This is usually physical, but often can be mental in the form of poor concentration or lack of creative energy.

- **Recurrent injuries.** Do you know many people who don't have any type of physical complaints? Shoulder and back pain, knee and wrist problems, weak ankles. It's not normal to have any injury at any age, even for people who exercise. When you have an injury, it means something went wrong, typically in the aerobic system and most often in the aerobic muscle fibers, and the end result is dysfunction in a joint, muscle, ligament or tendon.

- **Excess storage of fat.** When the aerobic system doesn't work effectively, the body stores more fat.

- **Blood-sugar stress.** The many symptoms include frequent hunger, cravings for sweets or caffeine, tiredness after meals, moodiness, etc.

- **Hormonal imbalance.** Premenstrual syndrome and menopausal symptoms are common in women with aerobic deficiency. But both men and women can develop hormonal imbalances, including low levels of sex hormones (discussed later).

- **Poor circulation.** Since so many of the body's blood vessels are found in the aerobic muscle fibers, a lack of aerobic function results in fewer operating blood vessels and diminished blood flow.

In addition, ADS is associated with an increased production of lactic acid. The body is always making lactic acid, and it's always regulated. But the combination of poor aerobic function and an overactive anaerobic system may result in too much lactic acid. This can not only further reduce aerobic function but also contribute to depression, anxiety, phobias and even suicidal tendencies. It's even been shown that raising lactic-acid levels in normal, healthy people can produce these symptoms. This is probably due to the effect of lactic acid on the nervous system. Excess lactic acid can also disturb coordination. It's a cause for concern, especially in athletes and others who require a more finely tuned, coordinated body for their work or sport. A high-carbohydrate diet, too much refined-sugar intake and a low-fat diet can also aggravate high lactic-acid levels, as can various nutritional imbalances such as low levels of thiamine (vitamin B1).

Other symptoms related to higher lactic-acid levels include angina pectoris, seen in patients with certain heart problems. The heart is a muscle, and it's not immune to the damaging effects of lactic acid. High levels of lactic acid create a major stress on the heart and blood vessels and may aggravate existing problems such as high blood pressure and heart disease. This may be one reason why the incidence of heart attacks in people who are running or jogging is relatively high — a combination of ADS and excess lactic acid. (It should be noted that anaerobic muscles normally produce lactic acid, and when entering the bloodstream lactic acid is converted to lactate.)

Optimal aerobic function is the foundation of fitness and another key to great human performance. And, as you'll see in the coming chapters, it's relatively easy to perform.

23

The Anaerobic Epidemic

Many people use the body's anaerobic system in an effort to keep up with the fast pace of a stressful life, often leaving the healthy aerobic system behind. Anaerobic muscle fibers provide us with the power and speed we sometimes need in the course of the day. When we see great athletes on TV or in ads, it's often their anaerobic qualities that we find so impressive — speed, power and big muscles. The problem is that many people seek out this type of body at the expense of their aerobic systems, and therefore their health.

In order to be both fit and healthy, anaerobic function must be balanced with aerobic function. Unfortunately, many who exercise are willing to improve their anaerobic systems even at the risk of losing aerobic function. Muscle machines, gyms with mirrors, and promises of "abs of steel" attract many customers. Bulking up has become analogous with health but often ends with poor health. Worse yet, we are educating our children to follow the same path by promoting no-pain, no-gain philosophies.

The anaerobic system includes the anaerobic muscle fibers, along with the related mechanisms used during high-stress activity. This includes increased sugar-burning, reduced fat-burning, and stress. While we can't survive without this mechanism, it's the imbalance that's the problem.

The imbalances caused by excess anaerobic function, physically developed through anaerobic exercise, can result frequently in injuries, illness, metabolic and hormonal imbalances, and added stress on the nervous system. You don't want to turn off this system, or neglect it; but balance it with the aerobic system.

Interestingly, the same type of imbalance can also occur in someone who is physically inactive. The out-of-shape person must rely on one of the energy systems, but because the aerobic system is not turned on, the anaerobic system becomes active to supply the energy needs. It's not unlike an overtrained athlete who builds the anaerobic system with too much hard work and too little aerobic exercise. In both instances the same type of imbalance occurs — too little aerobic and too much anaerobic activity.

Excess anaerobic activity, through some combination of over- or under-exercise, work stress or diet, inhibits the aerobic system through several mechanisms:

- Increased anaerobic function can change your muscle fibers, resulting in more anaerobic fibers and fewer aerobic ones.

- Increased anaerobic function produces more lactic acid which can inhibit the enzymes necessary for the aerobic fibers to function properly.

- Eating too much carbohydrate, especially refined sugar, increases the sugar-burning anaerobic system while decreasing fat-burning.

- Too much anaerobic function can be a significant stress, and, like any stress, can increase stress hormones to dangerous levels.

It's possible to improve both aerobic and anaerobic function, with the result of high levels of both. But the first step must be improving your aerobic system. Since the human body is made up of mostly aerobic muscle fibers, most of your physical activity should be aerobic. There is also a lifestyle factor to consider: For many people, from the time they get up in the morning until they finally drop back into bed at night, they are rushing, hurrying and continuously under stress. We need to learn to better pace our lives for the 1,000-mile journey. Aerobic exercise, along with good nutrition, can correct common anaerobic system excesses, allowing you to build better health.

Case History

Gary, a high-level executive in a stressful job, started exercising at his company's gym. At first he felt great. He lifted weights three or four times a week, jogged on the treadmill and played squash. But after a few months his shoulder began hurting. Then his knee started to hurt and he felt much more tired during the day, unable to concentrate on his work. My examination found Gary to be in a state of anaerobic excess. He was placed on an easy aerobic program of the same duration, with walking, easy stationary cycling and swimming, and was asked to do no anaerobic exercise. Within three weeks, Gary was much more energetic, and his shoulder and knee problems were gone. After three months of building up his aerobic system, Gary was ready to add weights to his routine.

Gary had to do two things to improve his fitness and health. First, he had to temporarily stop all anaerobic exercise. By doing this, a significant inhibiting stress was taken off the aerobic system. Second, he had to develop his aerobic system. In Gary's case, it took three months to build his aerobic system to a level that was balanced with his anaerobic system. Only then could he return to anaerobic work.

Anaerobic Exercise and Wasting Disease

Some people obtain important benefits from lifting weights or performing other hard anaerobic exercise, when performed in balance with aerobic function. However, for most people, ongoing anaerobic exercise creates a body state similar to cancer, HIV or other wasting diseases. Studies show that the biochemical changes seen in chronic disease states are similarly found in people who perform anaerobic exercise in as little as three times a week for one hour over a four- to eight-week period. The problems include low amino acids (such as glutamine and cysteine), low T-cell counts (from reduced immune function) and the loss of lean body tissue (muscle). Even in those who lost weight, it was found that most of what was lost was muscle, not fat. These same problems were not observed in aerobic exercisers.

Another problem associated with both anaerobic training and chronic disease is oxidative stress (discussed in a later chapter).

The significant production of oxygen free radicals can cause damage to virtually all bodily systems. This significantly increases the need for antioxidants, something of which most people don't get enough.

The time necessary to develop the aerobic system is sometimes referred to as building an aerobic base, and it's the foundation of your fitness. To do this efficiently, it takes time, about three months minimally, or for many people, up to six months or more. It takes discipline to not train harder than your aerobic system wants, thereby becoming anaerobic when working out, and to pay attention to all lifestyle factors related to improving the aerobic system. The majority of a yearly program should be made up of aerobic exercise, with shorter periods of anaerobic training, if any. Most people — from casual exercisers to highly competitive athletes — can obtain tremendous benefits from aerobic activity with little or no need for anaerobic training. Anaerobic athletes can carefully learn how to weave in sufficient anaerobic training without damaging the aerobic base. On the dietary and nutritional side, be sure to eat enough protein to meet the needs for glutamine, cysteine and other amino acids, with fresh vegetables and fruits for antioxidants, and take supplements if these nutrients are not obtained from the diet. For athletes, more details can be found in my other books on eating and training for endurance.

Lifting Weights? Do It Right

The various types of weight-resistant exercise, whether you use machines, free-weights or push/pull/sit ups, and whether you perform more or less reps, are always anaerobic. They can help you maintain strength and muscle mass, especially as you age. But incorporating this type of anaerobic training into an overall healthy conditioning program can be tricky. Start your weight-training program by doing none at all — first build a strong aerobic base as discussed in the next chapter. Walk, run, jog, cycle or perform other aerobic activity before introducing anaerobic training.

Once your aerobic system is ready to handle anaerobic exercise, you must determine how much it can handle. Everyone is different, and stress from all other areas in life should be a consideration as stress is like anaerobic exercise. For some people one anaerobic workout per week is sufficient; others with low-stress lifestyles may be able to handle up to three weekly anaerobic workouts.

For most people, the bulk of anaerobic benefits will be gained in three to four weeks, at which point it's time to focus again on the aerobic system. In this way you will be able to reap the benefits of anaerobic training with less chance for illness, injury or compromised body chemistry.

24

Heart-Rate Monitoring

Consistently performing aerobic exercise is a key to developing the aerobic system. You can walk, jog, run, bike, swim, dance or do almost anything aerobically. Unfortunately, these activities can also be anaerobic. You can take the guesswork out of your workout and be assured you're truly aerobic by understanding your heart rate.

Throughout this book I've talked about fat- and sugar-burning. I previously discussed measuring oxygen and carbon dioxide during exercise to determine the respiratory quotient (RQ), which indicates how much fat and sugar a person is burning. As accurate as this may be, laboratory testing for RQ is also very impractical for the average person. The best option — the most useful and least expensive way — to make sure your exercise is training the aerobic system is with a heart-rate monitor.

I began using heart rate monitors soon after entering private practice in the late 1970s. Today, many people use heart monitors while running, walking, dancing or riding a bike. As you attain higher levels of exercise intensity, your heart rate increases, and less fat and more sugar is burned for energy. Most importantly, the level of exercise intensity will dictate how your body reacts to that exercise session during the next 24 hours. Higher levels of intensity, and higher heart rates, train your body to burn more sugar and less fat, while easier exercise and lower heart rates do just the opposite. You can monitor this with your heart rate.

There are two ways to check your heart rate, by hand or using a monitor. Trying to obtain your heart rate by stopping to take your pulse is often very inaccurate. If you are just one or two beats off in a six-second count, that's a difference of 10 to 20 beats per minute! When you stop to take a pulse, your heart rate decreases rapidly. In six seconds, the rate may drop by 10, 15 or 20 beats per minute. In addition, even the light pressure used to take your pulse from the carotid artery in the neck can trigger a more rapid slowing of the heart rate. Besides getting an inaccurate count, you run the risk of fainting. Using a heart monitor is the answer to these problems.

The best heart monitors employ a strap around the lower chest and sense the heart rate by picking up vibrations of the heartbeat through the ribs. The heart rate is then transmitted to a watch worn on the wrist. They usually have an alarm that sounds when you exercise above or below your individually set heart rate.

Other heart monitor devices measure a distal pulse. These include monitors with sensors that attach to your fingertip or earlobe to pick up pulses. They are less accurate and not as convenient to use for walking or jogging, but may be useful for working on a stationary apparatus, such as a bike.

Heart rate monitors are simple biofeedback devices, telling you what's going on inside your body. In this case, the goal is to be aerobic to train your body's fat-burning system.

As a student involved in a biofeedback research project, I measured responses in human subjects to various physiological inputs: sounds, visual effects and various physical stimulations, including exercise. The observed reactions were evaluated by measuring temperature, sweating, heart rate and other factors. It became evident that using the heart rate to objectively measure body function was simple, accurate and useful. Its application in exercise was obvious. This information became important as I developed various biofeedback-based programs including treatment of muscle problems, improving brain function and individualizing exercise programs.

When I began using heart monitors to evaluate the quality of workouts done by patients, and correlated these observations with other clinical measurements of patients, it led to the development of a formula for determining the best heart rate to use for building the aerobic system.

The 180 Formula

The first step in the ideal exercise program is to find what level of effort is best for you. This corresponds to a particular heart rate, which, when not exceeded, will give you optimal aerobic benefits.

This is the 180 Formula, and it's been a solid, time-tested method of training the aerobic system in beginners, world class and professional athletes, and for the rehabilitation of many types of patients since the early 1980s.

Many people are familiar with the 220 formula, and others think the talk test works well. But neither are effective, and the 180 Formula replaces both.

The talk test assumes you are exercising within your aerobic range if you can comfortably talk to an exercise partner during a workout. This test is unreliable and in fact often maintains someone in a mild anaerobic state.

The 220 formula is still widely used despite its inaccuracy. You subtract your age from 220 and multiply the difference by a figure ranging from 65 to 85 percent. The resulting number supposedly provides you with an aerobic training heart rate. This formula contains two serious errors. It assumes that 220 minus your age is your maximum heart rate. In reality, most people who obtain their maximum heart rate by pushing themselves to exhaustion (I don't recommend you do this) will find it's probably not 220 minus their age. About a third find their maximum is above, a third will be below and only a third may be close to 220 minus their age. The second inaccuracy is the multiplier, which can range between 65 to 85 percent. This arbitrary figure doesn't consider a person's overall health or fitness. Do you use 65 or 75 percent? How about 80 or 70 percent? Without a more precise indicator, you are leaving your training heart rate to a very wide range, and your fitness to chance.

Rather than guess, it's best to use a formula that is not only more sensible, but has a proven success record and is more scientific: the 180 Formula. This method also considers physiological rather than just chronological age. To find your maximum aerobic exercise heart rate, there are two important steps. First, subtract your age from 180. Next, find the best category for your present state of fitness and health, as follows.

Calculating Your Maximum Aerobic Heart Rate:

1.   Subtract your age from 180 (180 – age)

2. Modify this number by selecting one of the following categories:

   a. If you have a history of a major illness, are recovering from any surgery or hospital stay, or if you are taking any regular medication, subtract 10.

   b. If you have been exercising but have an injury, are regressing in your efforts (not showing much improvement), if you often get more than one or two colds or flu a year, have allergies or asthma, or if you have not exercised before, subtract 5.

   c. If you have been exercising for at least two years and four times a week without any injury, and none of the above items apply to you, subtract 0.

   d. If you are a competitive athlete, have been training for more than two years without any injury, and have been making progress in both training and competition, add 5.

For example, if you are 30 years old and fit into category "b":

$$180 - 30 = 150, \text{ then } 150 - 5 = 145 \text{ beats per minute}$$

The result of the equation is your maximum aerobic heart rate. In this example, exercising at a heart rate of 145 beats per minute will be highly aerobic, allowing you to develop maximum aerobic function. Exercising at heart rates above this level can quickly add a significant anaerobic component to the workout, and stimulate your anaerobic system, exemplified by a shift to more sugar-burning and less fat-burning.

If you prefer to exercise below your maximum aerobic heart rate, you will still derive good aerobic benefits, but progress at a slightly slower pace.

Note: it always pays to be conservative, so if your resulting number is lower, it's also safer compared to guessing it may be a higher number.

The only exceptions for this formula are for people over the age of 65, and those under the age of 16, as follows:

For seniors in category "c" or "d," you may have to add up to 10 beats after obtaining your maximum aerobic heart rate. That doesn't mean you must add 10 beats. This is such an individualized category, getting assistance from a professional would be very helpful.

For children under the age of 16, there's no need to use the 180 Formula. Instead, use 165 as the maximum aerobic heart rate.

If you're used to exercising, when you first work out at your maximum aerobic heart rate, it may seem too easy. Many people have told me initially they can't imagine it's worth the time. I tell them to not only imagine it will help, but to understand how the body really works. In a short time, exercise will become more enjoyable, and you'll find more work is needed to maintain your heart rate. In other words, as your aerobic system builds up, you'll need to walk, ride or dance faster to attain your maximum aerobic heart rate. If you're a runner, your minute-per-mile pace will get faster; bikers will ride at higher miles per hour at the same heart rate; and so on.

Case History

Sally was very dedicated to her exercise routine. She went to aerobic dance class four mornings a week, and walked twice weekly with friends. But her time was not well spent, she thought, since her weight and body fat didn't change much in the two years she worked out. She also was very tired on the days she did aerobics. I asked Sally to wear a heart monitor during her aerobics class and when she walked. Not surprisingly, her heart rate exceeded 180 beats per minute during aerobics, and averaged 155 on her walks. But Sally's maximum aerobic heart rate was 140. Thus she had programmed her body to burn more sugar and less fat.

After seeing that she couldn't physically perform the aerobic routine during an advanced class without her heart rate going over 140, Sally went to an easier class where she was able to control her heart rate at 140. She also began walking on her own, at a much slower pace. Within a couple of months, Sally lost more weight than in the previous two years, and her work-outs now gave her energy. In time she was able to go back to the advanced aerobics class and walk with her friends while maintaining a 140 heart rate.

Using a heart monitor during weight training won't show that you're aerobic or anaerobic; you're always anaerobic when lifting weights or doing push ups, pull ups or sit ups. When wearing a heart monitor during weight-lifting, for example, your heart rate continues to increase as you lift the weight. But before your heart rate reaches its normal peak, your muscle has fatigued and you've stopped the repetition.

Once you find your maximum aerobic heart rate, you can create a convenient range that starts 10 beats below that number. Most heart monitors can be set for your range, providing you with an audible indication if your heart rate goes over or under your preset levels. Set yours at the maximum aerobic rate you determined. Most monitors also provide for a low setting, which could be 10 below the high. This gives you a comfortable range. For example, if your maximum aerobic heart rate is 145, then the low would be 135; set the monitor for a range between 135 and 145. It's not absolutely necessary to work out in your range — you just don't want to exceed it. If you're more comfortable exercising under that range, you will still derive good aerobic benefits.

Perceived Exertion

The 180 Formula applies to all activities (except weight-lifting and other strictly anaerobic training). At the same heart rate, different types of exercise require about the same levels of metabolic activity. So whether you're swimming, biking or walking, many physiological parameters are the same, and the 180 Formula applies to all of them. However, there's a difference in how you feel between different activities while exercising at the same heart rate. This is called the perceived exertion; it's a subjective feeling you have about how easy or hard the workout seems. Running at a heart rate of 140, for example, has a perceived exertion that's lower than swimming at that rate. That is, swimming at a 140 heart rate (given the same physical know-how) usually feels more difficult. This difference has to do with gravity stress. The gravity-stress difference between swimming and running is significant; there is very little gravity influence in the water, but gravity maximally affects your body during running. A lot of energy may not have to go into countering gravity stress in the pool but just the opposite is true during a run. Another way of looking at this phenomenon is that the heart rate during swimming is lower compared to running at the same perceived effort, since the stress level is diminished in the water.

Riding a bike falls between the two extremes of swimming and running, along with cross-country skiing, skating and most other endurance activities. In these actions, there is some gravity stress along with mechanical factors, which relates to technique.

Technique can influence the heart rate significantly. For the beginning swimmer, the heart rate is usually much higher. As your technique improves, you waste less energy and the same intensity (pace) results in lower heart rates. Looking at this another way, you need to swim faster to maintain your maximum aerobic heart rate.

The benefits of training with a heart monitor are many, and only with time and experience will you come to truly appreciate them. One other significant benefit of applying the 180 Formula to your exercise is the body's chemical response to exercise at a relatively lower level of intensity. Normally, the body produces oxygen free radicals in response to many stresses, especially anaerobic exercise. Too many of these free radicals contribute to degenerative problems such as inflammatory conditions, heart disease and cancer. Increased free radicals also speed the aging process. Exercising above your maximum aerobic level causes the body to produce large amounts of free radicals, even if you're only a little above the level. Using the 180 Formula as your guide minimizes free-radical production. Studies show that training at this efficient intensity is ideal when free-radical stress is a concern.

The MAF Test

Another important benefit of using a heart monitor is the ability to objectively measure your aerobic progress. Feeling good is one of the benefits of aerobic exercise. And feeling like you're improving is good too, but subjective. A very objective measure of progress is accomplished using the *maximum aerobic function test*, or MAF Test.

The MAF Test measures the improvements you make in the aerobic system. Without objective measurements, you can fool yourself into thinking all is well with your exercise. More importantly, the MAF Test tells you if you're headed in the wrong direction, either from too much anaerobic exercise, too little aerobic exercise or any imbalance that is having an adverse effect on the aerobic system (for example, from stress or poor diet).

The MAF Test can be performed using any exercise except weight-lifting. During the test use your maximum aerobic heart rate found with the 180 Formula. While working out at that heart rate, determine some parameter such as your walking, jogging or running pace (in minutes per mile), cycling speed (miles per hour) or repetitions (laps in a pool) over time. The test can also be done on stationary equipment such as a treadmill or other apparatus that measures output. If you want to test your maximum aerobic function during walking, for example, go to the high school track and walk at your maximum aerobic heart rate. Determine how long it takes to walk one mile at this heart rate. Record your time in a diary or on your calendar. If you normally walk two or three miles, you can record each mile.

Below is an actual example of an MAF Test performed by walking on a track, at a heart rate of 145, calculating time in minutes per mile:

> **Mile 1:** 16:32 (16 minutes and 32 seconds)
> **Mile 2:** 16:46
> **Mile 3:** 17:09

During any one MAF Test, your times should always get slower with successive repetitions. In other words, the first mile should always be the fastest, and the last the slowest. If that's not the case, it usually means you haven't warmed up enough, as discussed later.

The MAF Test should indicate faster times as the weeks pass. This means the aerobic system is improving and you're burning more fat, enabling you to do more work with the same effort. Even if you walk or run longer distances, your MAF Test should show the same progression of results, providing you heed your maximum aerobic heart rate. Below is an example showing the improvement of the same person from above:

	September	October	November	December
Mile 1	16:32	15:49	15:35	15:10
Mile 2	16:46	16:06	15:43	15:22
Mile 3	17:09	16:14	15:57	15:31

Performing the MAF Test on a bike is similar. When riding outside, the easiest method is to pick a bike course that initially takes about 30 minutes to complete. Following a warm-up, ride at your maximum aerobic heart rate, and record exactly how long it takes to ride the test course. As you progress, your times should get faster. Riding your course today, for example, may take 30 minutes and 50 seconds. In three weeks it may take you 29:23 and in another three weeks 27:35. After three months of base work, the same course may take you 26 minutes. Another option is to ride on a flat course and see what pace you can maintain while holding your heart rate at your max aerobic level. This works best on a stationary apparatus. As you progress, your miles-per-hour should increase. If you start at 12 mph, for example, following a three-month aerobic base you might be riding 17 mph at the same heart rate.

Perform the MAF Test regularly, throughout the year, and chart your results. I recommend doing the test every month. Testing yourself too often may result in obsession. Usually, you won't improve significantly within one week.

For those who walk, or do other activities that, over time, will not raise the heart rate to the maximum aerobic level, it's possible to do the MAF Test without using the maximum aerobic heart rate. Since it's usually too difficult to reach that heart rate, choose a lower rate for your MAF Test. For example, if you have difficulty reaching 150, your max aerobic rate, use 125 during your walk as the rate for your MAF Test.

Performing the test irregularly or not often enough defeats one of its purposes — knowing when your aerobic system is getting off course. One of the great benefits of the MAF Test is its ability to objectively inform you of an obstacle long before you feel bad or get injured. If something interferes with your progress, such as exercise itself, diet or stress, you don't want to wait until you're feeling bad or gaining weight to find that out. In these situations where your aerobic system is no longer getting benefits, your MAF Test will show it by getting worse, or not improving.

Phases of Aerobic Function

An important element of the MAF Test is knowing what is normal and what isn't. During your exercise program, you could encounter three different phases: progression, plateau and regression.

When you successfully develop your aerobic system, you will have more energy and better aerobic function, with corresponding improvements in your MAF Test. This is the progressive phase, and it can and should continue for many years without regression. As you improve, further progression will happen more slowly. For example, the first year your walking may improve from 18 minutes to 13 minutes per mile. The second year, your improvement may only go from 13 minutes per mile, walking, to 10 minutes per mile, jogging.

There will also be periods of plateaus. Actually, there are two different kinds of plateaus, one normal and the other unhealthy. With improvement, you will eventually arrive at a normal leveling off — almost as if your body needs a rest from the progress it's making. The metabolic, neurological and muscular aspects of the body require a period of adjustment, and the body may need some time for a recovery. These normal plateaus shouldn't last too long, perhaps a few weeks to a few months. Then, progress should resume, as measured by the MAF Test. If you stay in your plateau for longer periods, it may be abnormal.

An abnormal plateau is due to some obstacle that prevents progress. The MAF Test can help diagnose an abnormal plateau. Once your test has stayed the same for too long, the next step is to find out why. There could be many factors.

The most common reason for an abnormal plateau is stress. Remember, stress can be physical, chemical or mental. Typically, some lifestyle stress or stresses could cause your aerobic system to plateau. The weather may also be a stress that can halt progression.

Another common reason for an abnormal plateau is the food you're eating. Too much high-glycemic carbohydrates are the worst; not enough fats, poor hydration, or any nutritional problems can contribute too.

Even worse than not making progress is regressing. Indeed, that's just what happens if your plateau is prolonged — an abnormal plateau will eventually cause your MAF Test to get worse each time you check it. If this happens, your body is in a "red alert" and you should be very cautious. This is when you become most vulnerable to injury and ill health. One recommended strategy is to cut your overall exercise time by 50 percent until you find the problem. This will at least ensure you get more rest and recovery. If you don't respect the advice of your body, you may ultimately need to seek first-aid advice from a professional. Exhaustion, injury, illness or some other major breakdown, possibly including mental breakdown, can occur.

Factors That Affect the MAF Test

There are a number of factors that may affect your MAF Test results. When walking, for example, the type of track surface may have a slight influence on your pace. The modern high-tech track surfaces result in a slightly faster pace, whereas the old cinder and dirt tracks will slow your pace at the same heart rate. Uneven tracks will give slower times compared to perfectly flat surfaces. On your bike, the roughness of the road surface, varying grades and traffic can affect your test results. Hills usually result in a slowing of pace, unless there are significantly more downhills. A good option is to use a stationary apparatus on your test days.

To ensure the MAF Test is accurate, be consistent; use the same course or method each time you test yourself. If you change your test course, be sure to note it in your diary or chart.

Other factors that could affect your test include weather conditions such as wind, rain, snow, temperature and humidity; altitude; hydration; and your equipment. Most of these factors can work against you by increasing your physical effort, which raises the heart rate. Since you are working at a specific heart rate, the result is a slower pace.

One other factor worth mentioning is ill health. When you are sick, your body's immune system is working hard to recover, and it needs all the energy it can get. The last thing your body wants to do at this time is work out, especially when you have an elevated temperature. Don't exercise if you are ill. If you've ever attempted it and worn a heart monitor, you know what happens: your heart rate elevates, sometimes drastically. The same effect is observed if you are anemic: less oxygen can be delivered to the muscles, and your tests will worsen. For women, menses can also increase heart rate.

By using the 180 Formula and regularly performing the MAF Test you will be on the right road for improving fitness and health. But there's one more bonus — warming up and cooling down.

An Aerobic Bonus: Warm-Up and Cool-Down

Most people think that warming up means stretching. This isn't true. A real warm-up provides many important benefits, most of which stretching can't give. What's more, stretching can often do more harm than good.

Warming up aerobically is the first step of exercise; it's the slow shifting of blood into the working muscles. The key word is slow. Shifting the blood into the muscles too quickly can be a significant stress on the rest of the body. Specifically, the blood going into the muscles comes from other important areas of the body including the nervous system, adrenal glands and intestines. Diverting the blood out of these areas and circulating it into the muscles too quickly can be much like going into shock. When a warm-up is done slowly, the organs and glands can properly compensate for this normal activity. Warming up provides three important benefits:

- It increases the blood flow, bringing oxygen and nutrients into the muscles, and removes waste products.

- It increases the fats in the blood that are used for muscle energy.

- It increases flexibility in all the joints by gently warming and lengthening the muscles.

The warm-up can be any easy aerobic, low-heart-rate activity. Begin your exercise by slowly raising your heart rate from its starting point of say, 75 beats per minute. Slowly elevate the heart rate, over a

12- to 15-minute period, arriving at your maximum aerobic level only after 15 minutes. At this point, you can maintain your maximum aerobic heart rate until nearing the end of your workout, when you begin to cool down.

The Cool-Down

The final 12 to 15 minutes of your workout are also important; it's vital to slowly re-establish nearly normal circulation without "pooling" blood in the muscles. You want to re-establish the normal circulation in the organs and glands to begin the 24-hour process of recovery and obtaining the benefits from your exercise. This slow lowering of the heart rate from the maximum aerobic level back to near-resting level is called the cool-down. Carefully bring the heart rate back down by slowing down your activity. Attempt to reach your starting heart rate, which is often not possible — but at least get within 10 beats of your starting heart rate.

The following graph shows heart-rate changes in relation to time during a 45-minute workout — A: Warming up, B: Maintaining the maximum aerobic level of 140 , and C: Cooling down.

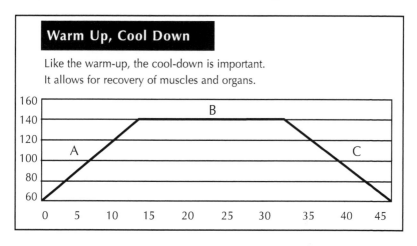

Warm Up, Cool Down

Like the warm-up, the cool-down is important.
It allows for recovery of muscles and organs.

Stretching and Flexibility

From your earliest years in school you were probably taught to stretch before exercising. Even people who don't work out sometimes think stretching is a good way to get rid of body aches and pains and so-called tight muscles. Go to any fitness center and you'll see that many people do it. Many think if they can touch their toes, they're fit.

There's very little, if any, scientific information demonstrating that static stretching is beneficial, especially the way most people do it. As a matter of fact, there's quite a bit of evidence showing it's harmful. One of the most common reasons people give for stretching is injury prevention. But studies show static stretching can actually increase the risk of injury! One of many examples given is the hamstring muscle group. It is both the most frequently injured muscle and the most stretched.

Many people need flexibility, and I often recommend that increases in flexibility be made to prevent injury and create a more stable physical body. This increased flexibility can be accomplished with a proper warm-up, rather than with stretching. Even patients with debilitating arthritis can improve flexibility with an easy aerobic warm-up of 15 minutes, and be as flexible as if they had stretched, without the risk. Before addressing the potential dangers, I'd like to talk about the two different kinds of stretching, referred to as static and ballistic.

Static Stretching

This is a very slow, deliberate movement, lightly stretching a muscle and holding it unchanged for up to 30 seconds. When properly done, static stretching promotes relaxation of the muscle fibers being stretched. But static stretching requires that each muscle group throughout the body be sequentially repeated three to four times. It also demands that the activity be done slowly. Note some of the key words: slow, deliberate, lightly stretched. And also note the need to stretch each muscle group three to four times. All this takes time and discipline, which most people just don't think they have or don't make time for. There are two different types of static stretching, active and passive:

- **Active stretching** is safer than passive and is accomplished by contracting the antagonist muscle (the one opposite the muscle you're stretching). For example, to actively stretch the hamstring muscles, the quadriceps are contracted.

- **Passive stretching** uses either gravity or force by another body part or person to move a body segment to the end of its range of motion or beyond — the reason this form of stretching can so easily cause injury. We sometimes see football players stretching one leg by having another player lean on it.

Ballistic Stretching

The second basic type of stretching is called ballistic. This is a "bouncing" method, and is the most common type done by both beginners and seasoned athletes. It makes use of the body's momentum to repeatedly stretch a joint position to or beyond the extreme ranges of motion. Because this method is more rapid than static stretching, it activates the stretch reflex, which increases tension in the muscle, rather than relaxation. This can result in micro-tearing of muscle fibers with resultant injury. Ballistic stretching is the type most people say they don't do, but really are doing. That's because most people are in a hurry when stretching.

Flexibility refers to the relative range of motion in a joint. This is related to the tension in the muscles around the joint, those that move or restrict the joint. The risk of injury is increased when joint flexibility is increased too much or is greatly diminished, or when imbalance in joint flexibility exists between left and right (or front and back) sides of the body (which usually corresponds to muscle imbalance as discussed later).

When it comes to flexibility, don't assume more is better. Studies show that the least flexible and the most flexible individuals were more than twice as likely to get injured compared to those whose joints had moderate flexibility.

People who stretch generally are injured more often than those who don't stretch. That's been my observation during more than 30 years of treating patients, and the opinion and observation of many other professionals in all fields. In addition, scientific studies support our observations. Halbertsma and Goeken, in a study of men and women 20 to 38 years of age with tight and stiff hamstrings, state that "stretching exercises do not make short hamstrings any longer or less stiff."

Richard Dominguez, an orthopedic surgeon at Loyola University Medical Center and author, also disapproves of stretching. "Flexibility should not be a goal in itself, but the result of . . . training. Strengthening the muscles around a joint naturally increases flexibility. If you can bend a joint beyond your ability to control it with muscle strength, you risk either tearing the muscles, tendons or ligaments that support the joint, or damaging the joint through abnormal pressure on it." Among the specific stretches Dominguez says are most damaging are the yoga plow, hurdler's stretch, toe touching and the stiff-leg raise. The types of injury created by stretching aren't associated with just the muscle being stretched. The tendons and ligaments associated with that muscle, and even the joint controlled by that muscle, are at risk.

There's also a chemical factor to consider. Repetitive exercise, such as walking, swimming, biking and other activities, results in the production of chemicals that increase inflammation. Adding stretching increases the potential for even more inflammation.

Many athletes stretch to help performance. But studies show static stretching doesn't improve athletic performance and may actually hinder it. For those who require a wider range of motion, proper stretching may be necessary. These include dancers, sprinters and gymnasts, but usually not most people doing aerobic exercise.

Case History

Randy began his morning with 10 minutes of stretching. The first 15 minutes of his bike workout was spent riding up hills from his house out of the valley. When he first used a heart monitor, his rate surged to 180 within five minutes. Randy couldn't imagine how any of that was related to his low-back pain. But by performing manual muscle testing, we discovered that Randy's hamstring muscles were overstretched, and therefore were not helping to support his low back. The first recommendation was to stop stretching his already overstretched hamstrings. Within a couple of weeks Randy's low-back pain improved. This was followed by the difficult task of adjusting his morning ride to include a warm-up, and to avoid going directly to the hills, with the resultant high heart rate. The solution was for Randy to ride indoors on a stationary apparatus for about 15 minutes before going outside, then riding very slowly until getting past the hills. When he was able to accomplish this, both his back pain and his chronic asthma disappeared.

Yoga and other "whole-body" flexibility activities are very different from stretching as I've described it above. When properly done, in a very slow, deliberate and easy motion, whole-body flexibility activities are healthy, safe and very effective. They're also recommended as a source of relaxation and meditation. If you wish to learn yoga or other flexibility activities find a course or an instructor who won't rush the sessions or push you beyond your limits. Don't attend if you can't put in the appropriate amount of time, and never go beyond your needs. Too many people try to rush into yoga positions that normally take a long time to establish.

25

Your Exercise Program

It's clear that regular aerobic exercise is essential for you to attain optimal fitness and health. But I want to re-emphasize that I'm not talking about a no-pain, no-gain exercise program that will fall by the wayside as quickly as you start it. Instead, incorporate into your lifestyle an ongoing, long-term natural aerobic exercise routine that will greatly improve your energy levels, stamina and endurance, while helping you tone the aerobic muscles and train your body to burn more fat for energy. Physical activity should be something that you look forward to continuing for a lifetime.

Exercise programs are quite individual. Some people just want to stay fit and healthy, and keep their weight in check. Others have goals such as training for the Ironman Triathlon. For either of these types, and for everyone in between, many basic principles are the same. All people who exercise want to gradually build up to a specific level, using the 180 Formula to improve aerobic fitness. Additionally, anyone on an exercise plan needs to balance this program with everything else in his or her life, including proper rest and recovery. I've trained many world class and professional athletes using these same principles outlined in this book; likewise for those just beginning. The volume of training is the difference. For serious athletes, training paces get significantly faster as their aerobic systems improve.

Walking Your Way to Fitness
Nothing is better than walking for overall fitness and health. Of all the types of exercise, walking is the one I recommend the most, and not just for beginners, but for regular exercisers and even professional athletes. It's the most fail-safe exercise. Scientific studies show that walking burns a higher percentage of fat than any other activity because of its low intensity. Walking activates the small aerobic muscle fibers, which often are not stimulated by higher-intensity aerobic workouts.

Walking also helps circulate blood, process lactic acid and improve lymph drainage (important to the body's waste-removal system).

Walking is one of the best ways to get started on an exercise program since it's a simple, low-stress workout that is not easily overdone. Walkers generally have little difficulty keeping their heart rates from getting too high, though there are exceptions. If there's a problem with walking, it's that the heart rate won't go high enough into the maximum aerobic range (which isn't absolutely necessary). The mechanics of walking result in less gravity stress than you experience jogging or running, but still enough to give you the important fat-burning benefits, and others such as bone-strengthening effects.

We've all heard and read about the many wonderful benefits of exercise. But did you know most studies that demonstrate these great benefits were done using walking? You don't need to make exercise complicated, expensive or intense. And I'm talking about just an easy walk — not power walking, race walking or carrying weights. Here are some of the facts about the benefits of easy walking:

- Regular, easy walking increases life expectancy. It also helps older adults maintain their functional independence, an important concern for society. Currently, the average number of non-functional years in our elderly population is about 12. That's a dozen years at the end of a lifespan of doing nothing: unable to care for yourself, walk, be productive or just enjoy life.

- Regular, easy physical exercise such as walking can help prevent and manage coronary heart disease, the leading cause of death in the United States, as well as hypertension, diabetes, osteoporosis and depression. This occurs through improved balance of blood fats, better clotting factors, improved circulation and the ability to more efficiently regulate blood sugar.

- Regular exercise like walking decreases your risk of developing degenerative disease. The lack of exercise places more people at risk for coronary heart disease than all other risk factors. Aerobic deficiency is an independent risk factor for coronary heart disease, doubling the risk. Inactivity is almost as great a risk for coronary heart disease as cigarette smoking and hypertension.

- Walking is associated with a lower rate of colon cancer, stroke and low-back injury.

All this can be accomplished with easy aerobic exercise. How easy? The equivalent of a sustained 30-minute walk, four or five times a week. Less than 30 percent of Americans are this active, including children who spend most of their spare time watching TV.

For some people, especially those who have been very inactive, very overweight or have chronic illness, even walking may pose overexercise problems. Whether 18 or 80, if you're beginning an exercise program, or have been inactive for a period of time and now want to start walking, consider using a heart monitor to take the guesswork out of your walk. I've seen too many beginners walking with too high a heart rate. It's often because they're with other people and the instinct to be competitive comes into play. Talking while walking also increases the heart rate, and so does walking up a hill too fast before some level of fitness has been achieved. Former athletes seeking to restore their fitness can benefit from walking; it keeps them from being too aggressive early in their programs. The most important thing for a walker to realize is that it's a fat-burning and endurance routine. Don't worry about speed; instead, concern yourself with endurance. Base your walking on time rather than miles.

Case History

Dave, a former college All-American, was in his middle-40s, overweight and feeling the effects of work stress. Since he was in the athletic-apparel business, he wanted to appear more fit. He began walking on the high-school track almost every evening. He got out of breath and tired easily, so he kept his pace relatively slow. After a couple of months with virtually no results, Dave asked for help. I told him to perform his walk as he usually does, but with a heart monitor. To our surprise, his heart rate exceeded 170 and stayed there for nearly the entire workout. Once Dave began using a heart monitor regularly and kept his rate at the prescribed level of 130, it was only a couple of weeks before he felt some positive results. And within a couple of months, Dave was thinner, had more energy and was walking faster.

Walking for the Non-Walking Competitor

Walking is also valuable to the competitive athlete whose sport may be cycling, running or any other more intense aerobic or anaerobic activity. Walking can be used as part of a warm-up and cool-down. Competitive athletes, when they're in a rush or working out with others, often don't warm up and cool down enough or properly. One way to ensure this is done is to walk for 5 or 10 minutes before each workout. Even if you bike or swim, a walk is a good way to warm up. The same is true for cooling down. When you get off your bike or get out of the pool, go for an easy walk to cool down. If you make it a habit, you won't feel right missing it.

Besides the cross-training effect on your muscles and nervous system, walking helps train muscle fibers you might not normally use in your workout. These are the very small aerobic fibers used during low-intensity activity. Many trained athletes say their weekly walk initially made them sore. That's due to the lack of use of these small muscle fibers, which also help break down lactic acid and bring more blood to the anaerobic fibers.

Walking is also a useful physical therapy following an injury or a period in which you have decreased your workouts for any reason. If you're injured, you may be unable to run or ride but have no trouble walking. Doing an easy aerobic workout is much better than doing nothing. And walking is a good way to come back from a period of time off without throwing your body back into high-level workouts.

Sometimes, even walking is difficult due to an injury or some other problem. Try walking in a pool in waist- or chest-high water. Gradually walk in shallower water before trying it on dry land.

As great as walking can be, many people feel uncomfortable about doing it. They somehow feel it's not enough of a workout, or it's too easy. It's that no-pain, no-gain feeling your nervous system has recorded in its memory. It's time to add some new memory.

Balanced Fitness and Health

Working out adds many new dimensions to your life — an important component of optimal human performance. Much like diet and nutrition, each person must find an individualized program to meet his or her particular needs. So start out as simply as possible. Then consider joining a group to get some psychological encouragement, as long as you can exercise within your own limits. Through this habit change, the exercise program becomes a positive addiction. Your routine will ultimately become a part of your day, like brushing your teeth.

There are a number of important factors to consider when starting or modifying your exercise routine:

- **Scheduling.** Create a realistic schedule of exercise that fits in with family, work and your other commitments. This will allow you to be more consistent, and help make it part of a new lifestyle.

- **Physical factors.** Be sure you can withstand the minor stress of exercise. Do you have some physical imbalances that may be aggravated by exercise? Take into consideration a history of prior injuries or conditions. Consider your workout surface — blacktop, wood and carpet are preferable to concrete, marble and steel. Grass and dirt surfaces may be safe, but they also can be stressful if they are uneven or too soft.

- **Chemical factors.** The proper nutrients, especially fats, are necessary for aerobic efficiency. High-sugar foods and drinks can be detrimental when consumed before workouts. Proper hydration is a must; drink water all day, not just after working out.

- **Psychological factors.** Studies have shown that people who exercise in the morning find it easier to maintain a regular program. But whether you exercise in the morning, midday or evening, be consistent. Write out a simple exercise program, if necessary. You are more apt to follow something you can see. Keep a log on a calendar or in a diary to see your success as the days, weeks and months go by.

- **Goals.** Set realistic goals. Some people merely want to progress to exercising 30 minutes a day. Be conservative, but don't hesitate to dream. Running a marathon after six months of training may be realistic only for very disciplined people who can control their stress. You won't break any records, and completing the marathon should be your only goal. I've worked with many patients who successfully, and in a healthy way, met that goal.

- **Habit change.** Starting an exercise program is, first of all, a change of habit. And as we all know, a habit change can be the most difficult change to make — even more difficult than the exercise itself. Generally, there are two barriers. One is just getting started and the other shows up two to four weeks later, when your enthusiasm wears off a bit. (Although being aware of this is usually incentive enough to keep you going.)

- **Time.** Most exercise should be measured in time, and not miles, laps or repetitions (except when performing your MAF Test). At the onset, a minimal time is best, since the purpose initially is to develop an exercise habit. The only exception may be if you progress to anaerobic workouts, such as weight-lifting, where a range of measurements should always be used. This gives you more choice, allowing for daily fluctuations in energy level and time restraints. For example, when using weights, the number of repetitions may be 10 to 15, rather than doing a predetermined exact number based on some program not meant for you.

- **Intensity.** The intensity of your workout is an important consideration, as measured by the heart rate. Make sure you understand how to find your maximum aerobic heart rate using the 180 Formula. Base your exercise program on time and intensity (as per heart rate); e.g., 30 minutes of walking at a heart rate not to exceed 140 beats per minute, five times per week.

A Word for Beginners

Even if you've never been active, aerobic exercise is easy and simple. If you are in reasonably good health and have no serious problems or injuries, it can be done with a simple 30-minute walk a minimum of four to five times per week. You can do this on your way to work, or on your way home, as part of your lunch break or anytime. It can be performed walking indoors or outdoors. Or you can use a treadmill or stationary bike, either in your home or at the gym. A simple aerobic workout will easily fit into your current work schedule and requires no special equipment, clothing or gear. Here is a typical starting program for a beginner:

- 30 total minutes easy walking.

- 12-minute warm-up period, 12-minute cool-down period.

- Heart rate not to exceed the maximum aerobic level.

- Monday through Friday schedule.

- Saturday and Sunday off.

You can always fit in a 30-minute workout at some point during the day. Within that time, include at least a 12-minute warm-up period, where your activity level is very easy. For the next 6 minutes move at a faster pace, but not so fast that it becomes uncomfortable — there's no need to break a sweat and you should be able to carry on a conversation. The remaining 12 minutes is your cool-down, another period of very easy activity. This is an optimal aerobic workout — one you can do in your work clothes during the course of the day.

Remember, your basic beginning program should be tailored to your specific needs. While most people are capable of at least 30 minutes of walking, perhaps 45 minutes is a good starting point. The maximum starting point for any beginner is an hour. Still others may benefit starting with 20 minutes per session. If you are recovering from a chronic illness, or have been very inactive all your life, you should consider only 15 minutes of exercise, or even 10 minutes, as a start, and also consult your doctor.

Case History

Alice was about to celebrate her 50th birthday, and thought it was time to get into shape. She was never physically active in sports, although she raised four children. She began a simple program of walking for 20 minutes, Monday through Friday, taking Saturday and Sunday off. After two months, Alice was ready to increase to 30 minutes each day, and after another two months progressed to 45 minutes. After a couple of years, Alice had the desire to take a couple of long walks a week, gradually working up to about 90 minutes each time.

How rapidly you increase the time period depends on your response. Whatever the starting point, assuming the proper time is chosen, maintain that time for at least three weeks. Listen to your body; it will tell you if and when you can increase. This is also true for any change: Maintain the new time for at least three weeks before increasing it if that's desired and there's no difficulty.

Don't increase more than 50 percent at any one time in a program of up to 45 minutes, and not more than 15 minutes when the program is 45 minutes or more. Some people are quite content remaining at 45 minutes. This is fine, since you can obtain many benefits when exercising at this level five times per week.

Perform the MAF Test every three to four weeks. If any problems develop, stop. A professional may be helpful in determining what's wrong.

What type of exercise should you do? When starting out, do almost anything, as long as it's aerobic. This may include, besides walking, riding a stationary bike, dancing, rebounding (trampoline), outdoor biking, swimming, hiking, cross-country skiing, and using various exercise machines, such as rowing and skiing. Jogging, or running, when done aerobically, is a healthy exercise. There is no universally accepted scientific distinction between running and jogging. For the purposes of this book, I refer to jogging when I mean a much slower pace. Running occurs with progression and more speed, and involves a slightly different gait. Any combination of these activities is also acceptable, as long as your heart rate doesn't exceed your maximum aerobic level. If you wish, do two or three types of exercise throughout the week, or even in one workout. For example, you can walk for 15 minutes, ride a stationary bike for 20 minutes and dance for 15 minutes. This "cross-training" routine is actually healthier than doing just one exercise each session.

Anaerobic activities, including any type of weight-lifting, sit-ups, pushups or activities that raise the heart rate above your maximum aerobic heart rate are not acceptable substitutes for aerobic exercise. They shouldn't be started until after you have developed your aerobic system. For the beginner, my recommendation is to wait at least six months, and for those modifying their program, wait at least three to four months before performing any anaerobic work.

Tennis, racquetball and similar sports often end up being anaerobic for the beginner, because of the type of muscle fibers used and the high heart rates produced. They're fun to do, but should be considered "games" and not exercise unless they're performed regularly; e.g., if you walk four times per week, play tennis once a week, or 18 holes of golf once a week. In that case, a proper warm-up and cool-down is important, as well as regulating aerobic and anaerobic levels.

Once you have progressed through a certain number of weeks without any problems, you may want to further develop your health and fitness. The following section is for people who wish to take their fitness to another level.

Progressive Fitness Programs

To further increase your level of aerobic fitness, you may wish to spend more time at or just below your maximum aerobic heart rate. Be sure to pay close attention to your heart-rate monitor to make sure you are not going over the maximum. If you can't reach your maximum aerobic heart rate by walking, you can jog or run, or perform other activities. Other types of aerobic activity, such as biking, swimming or dancing, can also be used to improve your aerobic fitness. Be conservative, and begin this phase slowly.

Case History

Kelly didn't like jogging, but wanted to do a variety of exercises. After walking regularly for more than a year, she joined an aerobics class. She continued to wear her heart monitor, walking three days a week and going to aerobics three days. After a few months, when the weather turned cold, she bought a stationary bike and rode it instead of walking, only venturing outdoors to walk if the temperature was tolerable. In time, Kelly had no need for her heart monitor; she only was able to get her heart rate to about 130 despite her maximum aerobic level being 145 beats per minute. She still performed her MAF Test, but at a lower heart rate. Kelly was very happy maintaining her activity at this level.

Basic Training

For many people, just exercising to be fit and healthy isn't enough. At some point in time this type of casual exercise program crosses over to a training program. Some people train to reach a certain goal, such as walking or running a certain distance or climbing a mountain. Others want to be competitive. While this information goes beyond the scope of this book, here are some basic training guidelines for those who wish to go beyond casual exercise:

- Take at least one or two days off per week for rest and recovery.

- Once per week, if time allows, do two workouts in one day, preferably one in the morning and one in the evening. Both should be relatively easy, below the maximum aerobic level.

- Once per week, do one longer-than-normal workout.

If after several weeks of building aerobic base your MAF Tests are continuing to show improvement, you may wish to add some anaerobic activity. Many people benefit by performing some anaerobic activity, as long as the aerobic system is well developed first, though for some with a high stress level, maintaining an aerobic schedule throughout the year works well. Anaerobic exercise may include lifting light weights, faster running, jogging, dancing, biking, or anything that raises the heart rate higher than the aerobic maximum. The following factors should be considered when scheduling an anaerobic workout:

- For most, one or two anaerobic workouts per week is sufficient.

- Anaerobic sessions should never be on consecutive days.

- Anaerobic workouts should be preceded by a day off, or a short, easy aerobic day.

- Anaerobic workouts should be followed by a day off, or a short, easy aerobic day.

- An aerobic warm-up and cool-down should surround anaerobic workouts.

- This anaerobic period should last no more than three to five weeks.

Caution!

Anaerobic exercise is a very common cause of injury, ill health and overtraining. It is also the most common reason so many who exercise have poorly functioning aerobic systems; they are anaerobic during many, if not most, of their exercise sessions. Be cautious when performing anaerobic workouts. Do your MAF Test during anaerobic periods. If you perform too much anaerobic work, you will know it by the results of your MAF Test.

Most people don't really need to do anaerobic workouts. Their lives have enough stresses that stimulate the neurological, metabolic and muscular systems to satisfy the minimal anaerobic requirements of the body. So don't be pressured into anaerobic workouts if you're not absolutely sure you want to.

An important rule is worth mentioning here again: Have fun in your workouts. If your exercise routine has become a stress, then something is wrong. Maybe it's time to change what you're doing. Maybe you shouldn't exercise with the people you're with. Whatever the case, if exercise isn't fun, find out why and correct it.

Aerobic Sex

One important and enjoyable function of human performance is the act of making love. Good aerobic function is a key ingredient for a good sex life. But for millions of people, poor sexual function is common. There are many physiological reasons for this, discussed below, and some that may be psychological (which go beyond the scope of this book and are not addressed).

In general, when you're fit and healthy, you should be physiologically and psychologically interested in sex. Specifically, a healthy aerobic system with good adrenal function (where many sex hormones are produced) plays a role in healthy sexual function.

If we look at the act of making love as a workout, we see a truer picture of what is happening. If one partner is always too tired in the evening, the problem often is aerobic deficiency. This may be caused by eating too many sweets or carbohydrate snacks in the course of the evening, or throughout the day.

Suppose the unresponsive partner isn't really tired. Perhaps that's the excuse used because he or she isn't especially aroused sexually. This aspect of lovemaking is, for the most part, hormonal in nature, and sex hormones are affected by stress. Estrogen, for example, plays important roles, from arousal to lubrication. Testosterone also plays a vital role in sexual desire. Excess stress, a low-fat diet or other factors can reduce these hormones and have a devastating effect.

It is no coincidence that complaints of a lack of interest in sex often coincide with high stress states. In many people, this "sexual deficiency" then contributes even more to the already high stress level, and prevents the person from getting a much-needed stress reduction. Sexual activity can be very therapeutic. In the course of your day and week, all kinds of stress can accumulate. That tension, the increased sympathetic activity often associated with stress, if not balanced, can be harmful. The act of making love, specifically, having an orgasm, can eliminate that tension.

What of the complaint, often heard from women, that "he never lasts long enough?" Among the factors associated with this occurrence is a lack of stamina. This translates to endurance, or the lack of it. The inability to endure sexually is another symptom of aerobic deficiency. Correcting aerobic deficiency often eliminates these complaints.

Another factor associated with the person who "doesn't last long enough" is that he is usually not sufficiently warmed up. Many people, more often men, choose to make lovemaking a sprint rather than an endurance activity. A slow warm-up of activity is vital to any workout, including lovemaking. In this instance, the warm-up is very important, and can be accomplished with foreplay. Spending enough time warming up will allow the hormonal system to properly evoke the normal, healthy response in both partners. Without a warm-up, you may not be ready to continue effective, enjoyable sexual activity.

Cooling down is another aspect of sex too often neglected, just as in exercise; it's vital to the complete workout. Like warming up, or foreplay, cooling down is essential and should include a slow winding down, with easy, light-touch activity that produces even more feelings of relaxation. Using exercise as a pattern, making love requires the same elements: a slow increase in activity, followed by the peak of the workout, and ending with a cool-down.

There are a variety of dietary and nutritional factors that can help sexual performance. No, there's no magic pill despite all the ads for such gimmicks. The factors that really work happen to be the same ones that help improve overall aerobic and hormonal function as discussed throughout this book. More importantly, there are a number of factors that can have a negative impact on sexual performance — the same factors that can inhibit aerobic function.

One aspect of sexual performance worth mentioning here is that of fertility. This problem can affect both males and females as potential parents. Women who want to conceive but are unable often suffer from a tremendous amount of stress. The first step for a woman who cannot conceive (after several months of trying) is to be sure that ovulation is taking place, and that intercourse is taking place at the same time as ovulation. This can be done using a kit available from drug stores. If that doesn't result in success, make sure both partners have been examined and all physical or chemical reasons have been eliminated. If there are clear problems, your doctor will most likely have some recommended therapy. If no clear problems exist, you may be on your own again, unless you are willing to undergo more extreme hormonal therapy. This type of therapy never made sense to me for two reasons: It's not very successful; and it's relatively easy to balance the hormonal status, often resulting in conception. If the more conservative approach fails, one still has the option to try more extreme measures.

The most common cause of infertility I have seen is carbohydrate intolerance, probably by reducing the important sex hormones estrogen and progesterone. Alleviating carbohydrate intolerance through dietary changes helps remove stress from the adrenal glands, which can increase DHEA and other sex hormones. Ultimately, this improves fertility, sometimes even in the most stubborn cases. (And sometimes when conception isn't wanted — so if you're of child-bearing age doing the Two Week Test — be careful.)

In the case where fertility takes place but maintaining pregnancy is difficult, similar problems may exist. The difference is in the hormones that are most deficient. In many cases of early miscarriage, progesterone is too low. The same dietary factors may be important, but in addition, a natural preparation of progesterone may also be needed.

Sexual function is a normal, natural and healthy aspect of human performance, one that should take place throughout life, not just during youth. Imbalances in the aerobic system or the adrenal glands can adversely affect the sex hormones, resulting in sexual problems. Many common side effects of aerobic or stress-related dysfunction, such as fatigue, poor circulation or depression, can adversely affect sexual performance as well.

26

Sports Shoes: The Danger Underfoot

Just like finding the proper formula for nutrition and exercise, it's up to you to find the right shoes for your feet. That may sound simple, but the truth is most shoes — even the ones in the impressive television ads — can be hazardous to your health. Most modern exercise shoes offer too much support, are too heavy, and have too-thick soles. What's more, many people are wearing the wrong size. The result is a formula for injury.

Biomechanically incorrect shoes can cause physical stress throughout your body, and contribute to injuries from the foot, ankle and knee to the hips, spine and other areas. Scientific studies show that the so-called protective features found in many shoes, including shock absorption and motion control, actually increase the likelihood of injury. For instance, some support systems can weaken your ankles, and soft, cushioned shoes can potentially lead to instability of the knee joint and other areas. Furthermore, the thicker the sole, the more unstable your foot and ankle become.

Many of these oversupported shoes are also overweight. The seemingly insignificant weight added to your feet, in the course of the day or workout, produces large negative effects in the economy of locomotion. For example, for every 3 ounces of shoe weight, a 1 percent increase in oxygen uptake is required for the same performance.

The soles of your feet have millions of nerve endings that sense the gravitational stress of standing and each step you take. This information is sent to the brain, which works together with your body to adapt to this stress by constantly adjusting your body during movement. This normal protective mechanism is meant to keep you from accumulating excess wear and tear, and from being injured. When you cover the foot with a shoe, you risk interfering with this adaptive mechanism by preventing the nerve endings on the bottoms of your feet from sensing and sending vital information to the brain. The more the foot is covered with thick, insulating materials, the more interference with the body's natural mechanisms. The result is a diminished ability by the foot and the rest of the body to adapt to normal activity, with potential damage to the ligaments, fascia, cartilage or bones in the foot. Because your feet are your foundation, any instability there could have dire consequences in the legs, knees, pelvis, low back or other areas.

The issue of impact is important, and shoe companies often infer their products protect you against this problem. But impact is normal; it occurs in the foot during walking or training whether a shoe is worn or not. Without a shoe, the body can adapt naturally to impact. With a shoe, there may be interference in that adaptation process.

Barefoot is best because there is no interference with the nerves that sense contact with the ground. Overall, those who are often, or always, barefoot have much fewer foot problems. For example, athletes who run barefoot are injured much less often than those who wear shoes. Unfortunately, this is not practical for most people, though you can still be barefoot whenever possible, such as in your home or backyard. And if you live near a beach or a grassy area you can also do some barefoot walking or running on these surfaces.

What to Wear?

The reality is that most people will have to wear shoes when going outside. When buying shoes, there are some things to consider. Look for shoes that are relatively flat and natural, ones that don't oversupport your foot or raise it off the ground too much. Many companies make these shoes, but in lesser numbers than the oversupported ones. In addition, a few running shoes called "racing flats" are built with less sole to come between your foot and the ground. Above all, forget the hype you hear about shoes. Consider the fact that one study of 5,000 runners showed that those using more-expensive running shoes with more shock-absorbing materials had a higher incidence of injury. It seems there is less chance of developing problems in less-expensive shoes. The main reason for wearing them is not support, but rather to protect the bottoms of your feet.

Excess heel height can also increase pronation, especially in shoes with heels that are thicker than about 1 inch. Too much heel height can also causes the entire body to move abnormally.

A significant problem with thicker heels and soles is foot strike. The natural running gait results in mid- to forefoot strike, depending on how fast the pace. But the thick soles used in today's running shoes, for example, forces you to land on your heels — this is not natural and a significant mechanical stress. Try running barefoot, and no matter how slow or fast you go it will be almost impossible to land on your heel. (Landing on the heel is a normal *walking* gait.)

In general, shoes with more cushioning are also likely to produce excessive pronation, a falling inward of the foot's inner, medial arch. This is especially true of shoes with added soft midsole material. Many shoe-support systems, including orthotics, can interfere with the normal functioning of the medial arch, the most important of three main arches in the foot. I have only on rare occasions recommended orthotics, and only for a short time while the cause of the problem was being corrected.

Sorbothane and similar materials commonly used in exercise shoes and after-market insoles can also be counter-productive. While tests on machines demonstrate Sorbothane's great energy-absorbing abilities, a study on humans shows that insoles made of this material actually increase leg stress by 26 percent, enough to cause stress fractures.

Beware: The muscles of your foot and leg, especially the calf muscles, have adapted to the thickness of your shoe. If you suddenly change your shoe style by wearing flatter shoes, your muscles may have to re-adjust their length. This may take a couple of weeks, during which you may experience some calf discomfort.

Sizing Up Your Shoes

A significant number of people are wearing everyday, dress or exercise shoes that are too small. In addition to foot problems, this can cause pain or dysfunction in the ankle, leg, knee, hip, low back, and at times as high up as the neck or TMJ (jaw) joint. And most often, the feet don't even hurt. A study done in my clinic over an 18-month period found 52 percent of all athletes were training in shoes that were too small. Once the problem was diagnosed, these patients usually required a change from one-half to one-and-one-half sizes larger.

Another study by orthopedic surgeons showed that 88 percent of women wore everyday shoes that were too small.

Case History

Jim had seen eight different professionals for his problems. Because his symptoms were in both knees, most of their therapeutic attention was directed there. But it was Jim's workout shoes that told the real story. His right shoe had an area where the large toenail had worn through. Upon measuring his foot, it was found that his shoes were one entire size too small. "I thought they should be snug," he said. After wearing the correct-size shoes for a week, Jim was able to exercise painlessly for the first time in two-and-a-half years.

You might think that the size of your feet is set by age 20, but that's not true. Normal increases in size, as a result of changes in weight, muscular imbalance or pregnancy, often occur regardless of age. Just being on your feet a lot can increase their size. This is due to the stretching or elongation of the ligaments and tendons, followed by a spreading of the bones in the foot. If you don't keep up with these changes by wearing larger-size shoes, you can create a major physical stress.

Wearing a shoe that's too small can cause a slow inward jamming of the toes, characteristically causing a backward subluxation of the first metatarsal joint, though any toe can be involved. This creates a mechanical instability in the foot which, if left uncorrected, can lead to other foot and ankle problems such as hammertoes and bunions. In time, the toes become spring-like; when a small shoe is slipped on, the toes spring in, and the tightness of the shoe is not obvious. The first metatarsal joint, however, is not as flexible as the joints of other toes, and therefore takes most of the abuse.

Due to the slow onset of this common problem, the first metatarsal jam is often asymptomatic; if you have it you usually don't complain of pain in that first toe joint. But visual examination of your feet will often reveal trauma, or micro-trauma (long-lasting mild stress) to the tips of the toes. This often includes discoloration of the nail bed (a darkened toenail), blistering or callousing of the toes, or swelling of the first metatarsal joint (the "ball" of the foot). In more extreme cases, inspection of your shoe will reveal wear and tear, inside and out, as a result of the nail or front of the toe trying to push out of the shoe, sometimes causing a hole in the shoe.

Looking inside the shoe helps diagnose the problem. If you have a removable insole, take it out and study it. Look at the wear pattern (especially the indentation made from the toes), and see if the areas compressed by the toes are not completely on the insert, as they should be. Toes that overlap the top of the insert obviously indicate a too-small shoe.

The importance of proper-fitting shoes can't be overemphasized. Here are some tips on finding an ideal-fitting shoe.

Always measure your foot when buying shoes. After a certain age, many people don't have their feet measured when buying new shoes, since they don't realize their size could have changed. As a result, the same shoe size is worn for years, or even decades.

Have both feet measured by a competent shoe-store salesperson, in a standing position on a hard floor. Do this at the end of the day, since most people's feet are slightly larger then, compared to the morning. (Of course, any meaningful daily size fluctuations must be differentiated from serious health problems, such as edema and certain pathological changes.) Use these sizes only as a gauge — the devices used for this measurement are consistent, but the sizes marked in the shoes aren't. A size 9 from one company may be more like an 8 from another. Don't buy shoes by their size but how they fit each foot. Even the same company may be very inconsistent when it comes to its own size standard.

Spend adequate time trying on shoes in the store. Find a hard surface rather than the thick soft carpet in shoe stores, where almost any shoe will feel good. If there's no sturdy floor to walk on, ask if you can walk outside. If this is not allowed, shop elsewhere.

Try on the size you think you normally wear. Even if that feels fine, try on a half-size larger. If that one feels the same, or even better, try on another half-size larger. Continue trying on larger half-sizes until you find the shoes that are obviously too large. Then go back to the previous half-size; usually that's the one that fits best. You may need to try different widths when available to get a perfect fit.

Don't let anyone say you have to break them in before they feel good — the best shoes for you are the ones that feel good right away. Even though you may develop the reputation of being a nuisance at your shoe store, your body will benefit. While many salespeople are aware of how to find the right shoe size, many are not.

For those who have a significant difference of more than a half-size between their two feet, fit the larger foot.

Many women fit and function better in men's sports shoes than in women's. The first rule, though, is that the shoe must fit properly. Some women don't fit into men's shoes, and some stores don't carry men's shoes in sizes that are small enough.

You may not find the right shoe in the first store you visit. Most outlets carry only a few of the many shoes in the marketplace. Often, shoes from mail-order outlets cost less. But be prepared to ship them back if they don't fit just right.

Remember, manufacturers design new shoes based on trends of style, color and fancy gimmicks to market the shoe. That's why shoe styles come and go. If you find the shoe that fits perfectly, buy several pairs. Just be sure to try them all on, since the same shoe style may vary in size.

Some patients I worked with bought larger shoes after their initial problem was diagnosed, only to find that their feet kept getting larger. At some point in time, they ended up with an increase of a full size or more. I have occasionally seen increases of two-and-a-half sizes over a two-year period in adults!

This situation is especially a concern for kids, whose feet always seem to be growing. When in doubt, get new shoes. Too expensive? Don't be afraid to buy some of the inexpensive shoes on the market. The $15 models wear just as long as the fancy ones for $150. Unfortunately, once kids see enough shoe commercials on TV, they may only want the expensive brands.

Actually, children should go barefoot as much as possible. When shoes are necessary for children, find them the best-fitting, thinnest shoes with the least support. And that goes for grown-ups too — don't be afraid to spend as much time as possible barefoot. It not only helps to correct existing problems, but also prevents common foot problems seen in many older people.

This information on the potential dangers of shoes is not new. The first published research to show these problems dates back to 1954; electromyographic studies demonstrated poor muscle function in the foot when shoes are worn. Modern shoes are even worse, as many newer studies continue to show.

"High-Tops"

Popular basketball shoes — "high-tops" — are promoted as a way to protect the ankles against injury. However, since high-tops were made ankle injuries have become the most common injury in the sport of basketball, where almost all athletes use this type of shoe. High-tops are also worn by many people who don't play basketball. And, like most commonly used "over-the-counter" supports, whether for the ankle, knee or other joints, they often weaken the muscles around the joint, ultimately contributing or even causing a chronic problem.

One study showed that during a two-year period, 78 percent of basketball players experienced some type of ankle injury. Of these, 83 percent were recurrent. Studies have not demonstrated that high-top shoes are able to prevent ankle sprains. In fact, Brizuela and colleagues (1997) showed that high-top shoes produced more ankle injuries. These same shoes also *reduced* the average jump height, and they increased the time needed to complete a short running course in comparison to those who wore low-support shoes — something to consider if you're playing basketball!

27

Self-Health Care

Most likely you're reading this book because you want to take more control of your health. The rampant problem of chronic disease, including the epidemic of overweight and obese people, now encompasses the majority of all the people in the industrialized world. As this problem continues to rise, no health-care system will be able to keep up with the medical needs of all these individuals. The health-care systems of all countries are already overspending while the explosion in costs has only just begun. The answer to the problem is self-health care.

There is a primary issue missing from the health-care discussions that come up at each election; an issue that would help ensure success and significantly reduce costs. If we are to truly improve the health-care system for the long term, each one of us must take more personal responsibility for health. Health care must have a primary proactive component — in which individuals avoid ill health and disease — instead of the current reactive approach where we wait for disease to occur then treat it.

Experts generally agree that most health problems, including most diseases, are preventable. In its truest definition, prevention refers to "outlasting disease" by being healthier at an earlier age. While "screening for disease" is important, it's a separate issue, and does not take the place of true prevention. As individuals, we are the only ones who can truly prevent disease.

Taking personal responsibility for health is a significant step toward improving the overall health of our own bodies, our families, our communities and the world. In doing so, health-care costs can begin to drop after year one, and dramatically be reduced further over time. The process is not unlike getting people to wear seat belts or quit smoking — both examples of true prevention. But the process must be expanded to include factors associated with chronic disease and ill health. These include the food people consume, levels of physical activity and stress.

How can we change a population's eating and activity habits? Much the same way that most people have been convinced to wear seat belts and smoking has been significantly reduced — with education. But that process cannot include lobbyists from the food industry and others who have conflicts of interest. There is a consensus of scientific and medical information that could serve as the foundation for education and recommendations.

The remaining chapters in this book continue the process of learning about fitness and health. They highlight some very important issues that put into focus the information from all previous chapters. This includes discussions about some of the problems people fear most — cancer, heart disease and poor aging, as well as the issues that are the causes of these and other health problems — stress, being overfat and chronic inflammation. These chapters also address areas of the body that are primary for physical, chemical and mental health — the muscles and bones, gut and brain.

Today there's a revolution afoot in the world of health care. Growing numbers of people are beginning to realize they must take personal responsibility for health. This revolution finds people shifting their efforts from crisis intervention to disease prevention. Instead of just regular visits to the doctor, these people are seeking information that can help them not only live longer but also enjoy a higher quality of life. Disease is not an unavoidable option for these people. The prospect of spending 12 completely dysfunctional years at the end of a lifetime is just not acceptable to them. In fact many people now rank longevity and quality of life as their No. 1 goal, and also recognize the enormously important role that diet, nutrition and exercise play in reaching this goal. I call this revolutionary movement self-health care.

In addition to longevity and quality-of-life issues, many people also are fed up with the expense of the modern health-care system. Health care is the single largest sector in the U.S. economy. In 2008, health-care spending reached $2.4 trillion, and is projected to exceed $3 trillion in 2012. This is 17 percent of the gross domestic product

(GDP), and more than four times the U.S. military budget. This cost is even more than other industrialized nations who provide health insurance to all their citizens (many of them spend only about 10 percent of their GDPs on health care). Despite this, the U.S. is ranked 37th, just above Cuba, in health care by the World Health Organization.

Without adequate changes, things will only continue to worsen. Baby boomers that today make up approximately 28 percent of the U.S. population will represent 67 percent of all those over 50 in America by 2010, posing even more challenges to the entire health-care system.

As the patient base grows, the "waiting for disease" model of health care will continue to fund an ever-expanding array of medical technology, devices and drugs enabling more patients to undergo more diagnostic procedures, take more drugs, see more specialists and be subjected to increasingly aggressive treatments. The advances in medical technology have increased the life expectancies of an increasingly large number of medically complex patients, many of whom require a high degree of monitoring and specialized care as well as rehabilitative therapy. However, this model of health care has failed and small numbers of health-conscious people are looking at real alternatives.

The cornerstone to promoting health, maintaining wellness and preventing illness is information that empowers individuals to assume personal responsibility for healthy diet and lifestyle practices, and the self-discipline to incorporate these practices into daily living. Despite this trend in the health-care system, the overwhelming evidence of the revolution toward self-health management is the increasing recognition and acceptance by the general public of the effects of diet, nutrition and lifestyle on achieving and maintaining optimal health and human performance.

Your Mission: Outlast Rather than Conquer Disease

Many experts point out that there is a maximum biological limit to aging. By shifting health-care strategy toward ongoing prevention rather than last-minute intervention, we seek to defer the onset of degenerative diseases to a point beyond the maximum age limit.

Health Care Failure

Almost everyone has a horror story about the health-care system, from procedures to insurance (not to mention the many scams in this sector). But when health-care fails to deliver, let's not forget our part. Health care can fail us when:

- We don't take responsibility by not taking care of ourselves. This involves eating exceptionally well; being physically active; significantly reducing environmental stressors (such as the chemicals in our air, food and water); controlling mental and emotional stress; and controlling body fat.

- We allow others to dictate our care — from insurance companies and employers, to the government and even our relatives.

- We don't have a health professional that matches our unique needs; e.g., you wouldn't go to a podiatrist for a sinus problem. Despite attempts to restrict our options by insurance companies, we do have a choice.

- We give health professionals free reign of our body and mind. We should work *with* health professionals in addressing our needs; they should also be our teachers, but we are always in charge.

- We cling to one particular health-care approach or philosophy and risk losing objectivity regarding personal health.

For example, an individual who is on a course of degeneration leading toward the onset of cancer at age 60 may be treated with therapies designed to delay the onset to age 130. If that person dies naturally at age 110, the onset of the cancer will have been avoided. This is "outlasting" disease. The result is a phenomenon called "squaring the survival curve," a concept promoted by James Fries of Stanford University, who says: ". . . many people with the early stages (of disease) never progress to the later stages during their lifetimes."

Delaying the course of what is known as the universal degenerative process means an individual need not expect a life of slow declines and failing capacities — as they often saw with their parents and grandparents. Instead, robust health can be maintained into old age. The bottom-line benefits? Better, cheaper and user-friendly health care. The National Science Foundation agrees: "Postponing universal decline would lower, strikingly, per-capita costs for older persons, starting with the 45 to 49 cohort. Chronic costs would be delayed and their duration reduced. Individuals would tend to stay healthy longer and decline more abruptly."

Many people are slowly dying of the very diseases they were led to believe could be conquered through research and development of new drugs while waiting for this idea to be realized. Along the way, quality of life crashes. The world is no closer to a cure for cancer, heart disease, Alzheimer's and most other killers, while we've known how to prevent and postpone them, in most cases, for decades.

A Classic Case History

All this philosophy sounds great, but is it real? Many in all areas of health care say yes. Let's look at an example of a person who is born relatively healthy, then falls into a long period of dysfunction with subtle but growing symptoms, ending with a diagnosis of disease. This case history is drawn from many cases I've read about and virtually a summation of most patient histories I've taken. This person is carbohydrate intolerant and will follow the current health-care model.

Some babies begin life with stress. Our future patient may have been adversely affected by being fed formula or sugar water shortly after birth, or by excess maternal stress. This stress, coupled with genetic programming (perhaps a grandparent was diabetic), may predispose the baby to develop a less-stable blood-sugar mechanism, adversely affecting the nervous system.

Within the first three years of life the baby's nervous, hormonal, immune and digestive systems develop significantly. Also during this time, psychological makeup is developed. The nervous system, at any stage of development, is especially vulnerable to periods of low blood sugar, sure to occur in this child. During the early years of life, a number of unhealthy patterns and physiological imbalances may develop. By age 10, this carbohydrate-intolerant child begins to develop symptoms. These include behavioral problems, various types of "learning disabilities," allergies, and asthma. If female, she may start to develop menstrual problems. As time goes on, intestinal symptoms and fatigue set in, and blood sugar may remain unstable. Some experts have linked blood-sugar problems to drug use and criminal activity. If brought to the attention of a mainstream medical doctor, he or she would probably rule out disease, and conclude that the problem may be psychological. Perhaps counseling would be recommended.

Before reaching age 20, this person — now somewhat overfat — attempts to lose weight through dieting. This vacillates from starving to lowering fat intake, accompanied by increased consumption of carbohydrates. It begins the process of yo-yo dieting, in which a lower caloric intake decreases metabolism, which results in some short-term weight loss, with the final consequence of weight gain.

To this point, this person would probably not have sought traditional health care for these seemingly minor but annoying problems. Over-the-counter drugs and other remedies provide symptomatic relief; effective marketing strategies promise help is just a pill away.

By the second through third decade of life, the carbohydrate-intolerant person usually becomes a patient. And at this point, many of the symptoms have worsened: fatigue, intestinal bloating and decreased concentration. Addictions to sweets, caffeine, alcohol, tobacco or other drugs are quite possible.

Many symptoms are now observable and measurable. Dizziness, caused by a significant blood-pressure drop upon standing, is common. Blood pressure may begin to elevate. Abnormal glucose-tolerance tests are sometimes found, but more often still appear normal. Other signs include increased fat stores, especially in the upper half of the body. Blood fats, especially triglycerides but also cholesterol, may begin to increase. More common and difficult to measure early is a clogging of the arteries with fat.

If seen by a traditional doctor, the patient may be put on a diet to help relieve the symptoms. This diet may be high in carbohydrates, and low in fat, red meat, eggs and cheese. And the symptoms just get worse.

Exercise is sometimes recommended. But with no direction, the patient frequently exercises too intensely in the hope of burning more calories. This leaves this patient worse off, usually with a more pronounced aerobic deficiency.

Soon after this stage, around the fifth decade of life, measurable pathological, or disease states appear. They may include high blood pressure, high blood fats (triglycerides and/or cholesterol) and problems handling blood sugar. These signs may now be accompanied by named diseases: hypertension, hyperlipoproteinemia and diabetes. There is now a very high risk for coronary artery disease and if fat accumulates, blocking the flow of blood to the heart, bypass surgery may be the only way to prevent death. At this stage, conservative measures such as exercise, diet and nutrition require more stringency to be effective, but still can play a major role in therapy. If disease is too advanced, more extreme countermeasures may be needed, such as surgery.

The last stage of life, the so-called golden years of the 60s and up, can literally be quite painful for both patient and family, and a great expense for all, including society. Our patient, now a medicated, hypertensive, overweight diabetic on the verge of requiring bypass surgery, remains at high risk until the end. But modern medicine has helped lengthen the life span. When death comes, it comes not only with pain and suffering, but also with great expense.

Could this scenario be changed? Could the suffering and expense be prevented? Clearly the answer is yes. And it's not just a philosophy. We can see it in action in people who follow the right path towards fitness and health.

Treating Functional Illness

Recognition of functional illness early in life, when it's more easily and inexpensively treated with conservative measures, including lifestyle changes, is one of the keys to self-health care. This is the true meaning of prevention. In medicine, prevention is thought of as a screening process, such as "screening for cancer" to find it early when it's more treatable. I prefer to think of prevention as postponing that cancer and not allowing it to progress to a diagnosis during your lifetime.

We are not fated to live and die with a game plan we don't control. We can alter the quality of our lives, and influence the quality of our children's lives. In these later chapters about managing our fitness and health — self-health care — I discuss many topics regarding dysfunction and disease and how you can take a proactive approach to true prevention. By effectively managing your own health you may not only be able to avoid disease, but also limit your exposure to the health-care system, attain greater quality of life and reach the finish line of your life journey in good health rather than in dysfunction. The most powerful tool you have in this quest is real information that works, and is user-friendly. The only thing left for you to do is embody this information by applying it to your own self-health care strategy.

Finding a Health-Care Professional

The concept of self-health care is fairly straightforward: You manage your own health. But sometimes along life's journey you need advice or treatment. This is when finding a good health-care professional may be helpful.

Good health-care professionals are in great demand because there are too few of them. The first thing to do when seeking a health-care professional is to ask around. Mention to your friends or relatives that you're looking for a certain type of health-care professional. This may be a nutrition-oriented practitioner, massage therapist, chiropractor, medical doctor or any number of different professionals with various expertise. A good place to start is with what used to be called a "general practitioner," now called a family physician. He or she may be a medical doctor, osteopath or other professional who is knowledgeable in treating the whole person. If more specific care is needed, this person should also have the ability to refer you to a specialist.

Once you have a name you can find out more by talking with current patients. Find out what they like and dislike about the professional they see. The important questions include those about how much time is spent on typical visits, if questions were adequately answered, and if the professional took the time to treat the person as an individual rather than a number. Also seek out information about philosophical compatibility — you don't want to work with someone who is opposed to how you have chosen to live your life.

Before making an appointment, don't be afraid to call a professional's office for information about how he or she practices. This is not unlike an interview: You want to know about someone before developing a professional relationship.

Once you make an appointment, take note of how this practitioner addresses your needs and concerns. If you have a good feeling about your visit, plan another as necessary. But if you don't feel comfortable, whether you can explain it or not, search for another health professional. It may take some time to find a person that best matches your particular needs.

One problem with our current health-care system is that by going to see a particular doctor or other professional, you're most likely only going to get that person's specialty as treatment. For example, if you visit an acupuncturist, you'll get acupuncture; visit a surgeon, you often get surgery; visit a dietitian, you'll get diet advice. But what if you have both surgical and nutritional needs for the same problem? It's uncommon to find a practitioner who can address all your needs, or who will refer you to another specialist, although these health-care professionals do exist and are worth seeking out. This is why you must actively manage the entire process. It's up to you to find the best health-care practitioners that match your needs. In my practice I performed a variety of therapies, but most importantly took sufficient time to assess the patient using a variety of forms (sent to the patient ahead of time), past medical records, diet analysis, a long oral history and a physical examination. An effective assessment is a key to successful treatment. My therapies included various forms of neuromuscular biofeedback, individualized diet and nutrition recommendations, stress management, exercise guidelines and others.

And finally, finding a health-care professional who is fit and healthy is very important.

28

Brain Power

To paraphrase the great singer-songwriter Bob Dylan, if we're not busy being born we're busy dying. This sums up the remedy for optimal brain function throughout life. Unfortunately, too many people start dying at a very early age.

It's estimated that one in four people in the United States suffers from some form of mental or emotional disorder. Many more have diminished brain function, which is often transient. Human error is a common result of diminished brain function, and the cause of the majority of automobile, airplane, rail, boating and other tragic accidents reported in the popular press every day. Medical mistakes, which kill and maim millions of people, are also usually due to human error. Whether it's poor memory, such as not remembering that phone call you wanted to make, or getting lost in your own neighborhood due to a serious cognitive condition such as Alzheimer's, most cases of these problems are preventable through proper food and nutrition, stress regulation and lifestyle. And, the problem isn't just about avoiding cognitive problems — you want your brain to function at a high level until you die!

Do you remember where you were when President Kennedy was assassinated? Maybe you hadn't been born yet. How about when the space shuttle Challenger exploded? Or when the World Trade Center collapsed? Most people have vivid memories of where they were when these intense events occurred. At the same time, many people can't recall a simple five- or seven-digit phone number, for example, or the name of someone they just met. The memory of traumatic events is so clear because the powerful adrenal response provides optimal blood sugar levels. It's also possible to harness this great and valuable function of the body and brain through proper diet and nutrition.

Your Brain on Blood Sugar

There's nothing magical about it, learning, memory, and all other cognitive functions have an undeniable relationship with stable blood sugar. Whether you're healthy or not, blood-sugar irregularities can hit you at any time, adversely affecting brain function.

While the body utilizes both fat and sugar for energy, the brain is primarily dependent upon sugar. If the level of blood sugar rises too much, or falls too low, the brain has an immediate reduced capacity. This means you don't remember as well, don't respond as well to external stimuli, and can't learn as easily. Reductions in overall mental performance can follow. From early in life a child's poor learning can be a problem. As adults we joke about "brain damage." In older adults cognitive dysfunction such as Alzheimer's disease is on the rise. Creativity, in both children and adults, is another mental process that can be compromised when blood sugar is not balanced.

As I have discussed in detail throughout this book, blood sugar is controlled by a number of factors, especially food, nutrition, exercise and stress. Here's a quick review:

- High-glycemic carbohydrates, especially sugar and processed flour products, can reduce and impair brain function due to the effects of insulin. The application of this fact is simple: Don't go to work or send your kids to school after a breakfast of high-glycemic cereal or other sweets. Most adults know not to drink and drive, but many still go to work, operate vehicles or embark on other activities that require optimal brain function without the right fuel.

- Blood sugar can be controlled exceptionally well by snacking on healthy items. By eating five or six meals daily you can help stabilize blood sugar, allowing the brain to do its job properly.

- Stress can wreak havoc on blood sugar and reduce brain function (stress is discussed in more detail in Chapter 31).

- Physical activity can help improve brain function in many ways. Aerobic exercise can help improve blood-sugar regulation and blood flow, control stress and influences overall brain function.

Brain Pain

When we consider mental energy, it's clear thinking and creativity we want, rather than that foggy feeling or depression. When you have a thought or feel a sensation from the outside world, it's the result of major chemical reactions in your brain. Billions of messages are sent throughout the brain and the nerves on a regular basis by brain chemicals called neurotransmitters. Different neurotransmitters make you feel different ways: high, low, sleepy, awake, happy and sad. Sometimes the brain may have too many of one type of neurotransmitter or not enough of another. As a result, you may feel too high or low, or too sleepy. A common end-result symptom may be depression or anxiety. When these problems develop, antidepressant drugs are sometimes prescribed to manipulate brain chemistry in hopes of balancing neurotransmitters and relieving symptoms.

For most people, diet can have a profound effect on brain chemistry, often as much effect as drugs but easier to regulate and without side effects. What you eat, or don't eat, for dinner can influence your sleep, your dreams, and how you feel upon waking. And what you eat, or don't eat, for breakfast can determine your human performance for the day.

Most of the 40 or more types of neurotransmitters are made from amino acids derived from the protein in your diet. Certain vitamins and minerals are also required for their production, including vitamin B6, folic acid, niacin, iron and vitamin C. There are many important neurotransmitters related to mental function. They include serotonin and norepinephrine — the two most commonly discussed substances. Let's look at how a traditional meal affects most brains, and why the confusion surrounding this issue continues.

Most people think getting sleepy after Thanksgiving dinner is due to the turkey — more specifically, the tryptophan content of the turkey that can sedate the brain. Tryptophan, an amino acid that can produce a sleepy feeling when consumed in high amounts, is relatively high in turkey. But while this notion is promoted year after year in the media, it's completely false.

The reason so many people get sleepy after Thanksgiving dinner — like many other meals and snacks — is not caused by eating turkey, but rather by eating all the trimmings made from refined carbohydrate and sugar. In the case of a typical holiday meal, it's the bread, potatoes (including sweetened sweet potatoes), gravy (made with flour), cranberries (sweetened with sugar), and of course those extra servings of pie (there's always more than one type to taste). Throw in some alcohol and it's no wonder you're craving more than just one pot of coffee.

While turkey does have a high amount of tryptophan, it has many other amino acids that prevent tryptophan levels from elevating in the blood (thereby not affecting the brain). The foods that reduce brain function the most are the carbohydrates which cause a rise in a brain neurotransmitter, serotonin — this has a calming, relaxing, sedating effect on the brain, with the more carbohydrates you eat, the more sedating its action.

Sleepiness after any meal may be indicative of carbohydrate intolerance. So if you often feel this way, it's time to evaluate, or re-evaluate your eating habits as I discussed in the chapters on carbohydrates. High-carbohydrate foods cause the brain to produce more serotonin. The individual who is easily agitated or mentally overactive may benefit from a meal with natural carbohydrates that are not high-glycemic. Too many carbohydrates, however, can produce too much serotonin in many people, causing oversedation or even depression. If you're a student, executive, or just want to use your brain better, you might find that eating sufficient carbohydrate to adversely affect brain chemistry is counterproductive.

While sweets are traditionally thought of as providing energy, they are in actuality mentally sedating. Sometimes sweets may give the feeling of a pick-up, but that is very short-lived, until insulin lowers the blood sugar, resulting in more fatigue.

If you need a mental pick-up, try eating some protein. A protein-based meal with little or no carbohydrates causes your body to produce less insulin, and provides a higher amount of tyrosine and increased norepinephrine levels. This neurotransmitter has a stimulating effect on the brain. The person who needs a mental pick-up or who gets sleepy after a meal could benefit from eating a high-protein meal with little or no carbohydrate.

Drugs are often prescribed to balance brain chemistry. Depressed patients are given medication to restore balance to the neurotransmitters. Prozac, Elavil, Buspar, Aventyl, Tofranil and Zoloft are antidepressants that affect the balance of serotonin and norepinephrine. (Tranquilizers, such as Valium and Ativan, have a different function and affect other neurotransmitters.) But these medications have side effects, including reductions in glutathione, the most powerful antioxidant that protects the brain from damage.

Brain Function and EPA

One of the most important brain nutrients is the omega-3 fat EPA (along with DHA). Most people won't get enough from food, so supplementation is often necessary. The omega-3 fats are key ingredients for the development and repair of the brain, especially the eyes. Imbalances in essential fatty acids — particularly deficiencies in omega-3 fats — have been implicated in depressive disorders in adults and behavioral problems in children and adolescents, including Attention Deficit Hyperactivity Disorder, difficulties with learning, impulsivity, hyperactivity, aggression and anger.

Researchers continue to identify the positive effects of EPA on the brain and also have established a direct link between an imbalance in fatty acids and depressive disorders. In fact, it appears that these fats regulate neurotransmitters in ways that mimic the effect of some antidepressant medications. These fats coat the brain-cell membrane, serving a protective function when neurotransmitters are fired in the synaptic phase.

EPA and DHA have other benefits in brain function as well. They are most vital for the fetus and child during development of the brain. They may also help control the release of the stress hormone cortisol, resulting in improved brain function. And, they may help reduce the severity of degenerative brain diseases that lead to memory loss and dementia, including Alzheimer's disease.

Other Brain Requirements

The brain's 200 billion cells also have numerous nutritional requirements for good function. These include a number of vitamins and minerals, and most importantly, water. Any dietary inadequacy can potentially have a dramatic impact on brain function. Numerous neurological symptoms have been associated with a deficient diet, including aggression, learning disabilities, depression, hyperactivity and memory problems.

There is an important relationship between folate levels and depression. Numerous studies show that many people with depression also have low levels of folate. Consuming foods containing this nutrient can significantly improve depression in these people. For this reason, anyone considering antidepressant medication should first be screened for folate levels through a blood test for homocysteine, the best indicator of folate levels in the body. For depressed individuals who have low folate levels, adequate folate intake and utilization may be as effective as Prozac or other antidepressant drugs for treating mild, moderate and severe depression. Folate is contained in green, leafy vegetables and fruits; in some cases, fruit, especially citrus, can be a better source than leafy vegetables. For many people, synthetic folate, or folic acid, from most supplements may not be as effective or as well utilized as folate obtained from real food sources.

Other micronutrients are important for the brain too:

- Sodium, potassium, magnesium and calcium are also important for sending messages through the brain.

- Iodine has an important role in brain maturation, beginning in the fetus soon after conception.

- In children, a strong association has been made between iron deficiency and Attention Deficit Hyperactivity Disorder.

- Zinc is important for growth and maturation of the brain and is used for many chemical reactions in the brain, especially those related to behavior.

- Copper is also related to growth and maturation of the brain. While copper deficiency has been associated with deterioration of mental function and physical coordination, too much of this mineral can have the same results.

- Manganese, like copper, is both important for proper brain function and has potential for adversely affecting the brain if taken in excess.

- Lead, arsenic and mercury are all toxic to the brain and pose real health problems throughout the world. Lead poisoning has been known for centuries. For years scientific literature has described mercury poisoning, ranging from contamination of fish through accumulated methyl mercury (introduced to the food chain by industrial waste) to consumption of grain treated with mercury fungicide. The debate over dental fillings is still a concern to many in the scientific community.

- Vitamin B6 is another important brain nutrient, and is used in the regulation of certain neurotransmitters. Because estrogen can reduce the levels of vitamin B6, this may be important for some women, especially those taking birth-control pills and on estrogen-replacement therapy.

Though caffeine isn't considered a nutrient, it is a drug with potential brain effects. This is obvious to those who regularly consume caffeine. One main effect is increased mental performance and alertness, though negative brain effects can appear soon afterwards when the drug wears off and you crave more, especially if your food intake is not adequate. The physical side effects of caffeine can be unhealthy for some while others can tolerate relatively small amounts of caffeine each day. It's up to you to determine if your body can tolerate caffeine, and if so, how much.

As you can see, a variety of dietary and nutritional factors can help improve brain power — beginning at fetal development and continuing throughout your life and into old age. Both children and adults can improve their brain function by choosing foods that match their needs. For example, eating a balanced ratio of protein, unrefined carbohydrate and fat can help optimize blood sugar, thereby improving cognition, learning and memory. Certain dietary supplements can also be very helpful, especially EPA. Making dietary choices that ensure proper nutrient intake, such as adequate folate levels, can also be helpful in regulating brain function and improving conditions such as depression. In addition to these dietary considerations, another factor that can improve brain function is proper management of stress levels.

In addition to nutrition, hormone balance is important for brain function too. In particular, sex hormones. They help regulate protein balance in the brain. Sex hormones are part of the big picture of hormone balance and stress discussed in more detail in Chapter 31.

Ritalin Works Just Like Cocaine

Scientists have found that Ritalin acts just like cocaine by chemically manipulating the brain's dopamine system to reduce distraction and increase attention signaling.

Ritalin was one of the first in what would become a group of drugs used to treat ADHD and related behavioral problems. These drugs are prescribed to millions of children. Many adults also take the drug, along with untold numbers of illicit users.

Like cocaine, Ritalin is classified as a Schedule II controlled substance by the Drug Enforcement Administration. It is among the most addictive and abused prescription drugs.

Despite its widespread use, Ritalin does not address the cause of the problem, but merely offers symptomatic relief. The side effects of Ritalin are numerous and include decreased appetite, which can adversely affect the child's nutritional state, as well as retarded growth, insomnia, increased irritability and rebound hyperactivity when the drug wears off.

In addition, while ADHD is often associated with abnormal brain chemistry, it is important to note that these types of behavioral problems often have other contributing factors, including psychological dynamics and social stress.

Psychotropic drugs have a reported effectiveness rate of about 75 percent. However, the effectiveness of natural remedies that include the use of dietary supplements and diet modification is also reported in scientific studies to be about 75 percent.

Children diagnosed with ADHD have been found to have low levels of omega-3 fats in their cells. Omega-3 fatty acids — particularly EPA and DHA — are key components in the brain and are central to neurological function and visual acuity. Studies show low omega-3 levels correlate with poor behavior scores and teacher scores of academic abilities.

This is due not only to lack of omega-3 fats in the diet, but may also be the result of having trans fats in the diet, which could displace omega-3 fats in cells. Trans fats come from hydrogenated and partially hydrogenated oils found in many food products, especially junk food. In addition, excess intake of omega-6 fats from common vegetable oils can result in low omega-3 levels in the body. Since most children don't eat foods containing omega-3 fats, taking an EPA fish oil supplement may be essential.

A variety of over-the-counter and prescription drugs can impair brain function. Many of these drugs won't give obvious symptoms that your brain is adversely affected. Alcohol can depress brain function, although in small amounts it can improve social activity — this may be a great thing for the brain. Balance is key — if a small amount of alcohol makes you feel bad after drinking it, especially if you don't feel right the next morning as well, it's best avoided.

Brain Waves
The brain generates electrical activity that when measured results in waves of different frequencies and amplitudes depending upon the level of consciousness, balance of neurotransmitters, and overall normal or abnormal function. Sensation, attention (self-awareness), intellectual activity and the planning of physical movement have distinct electrical correlates in the brain that can be measured with a device called an EEG (electroencephalogram).

There are four commonly measured brain waves, associated with specific states of consciousness:

- **Beta waves** (12-32 Hz) are associated with full awareness and a busy brain, such as during a business meeting, planning a trip or multitasking.

- **Alpha waves** (8 -12 Hz) are associated with a sense of "relaxed alertness" and high creativity, typical during meditation, listening to music, and when eyes are closed. The ability to generate alpha waves is associated with the self-regulation of stress and may contribute to an expanded state of consciousness.

- **Theta waves** (4-8 Hz) are seen in the awake but dreamy state common just before the onset of sleep. These waves are most prevalent in youth but occur during deep creativity and meditation in adults at any time.

- **Delta waves** (0.5-4 Hz) are very slow waves occurring during most stages of sleep, but abnormal if occurring while awake and may indicate a lack of adequate blood sugar or oxygen, medication side effects, or poorly functioning neurons due to nutritional problems or illness.

The brain should make specific waves in certain brain regions at appropriate times. An abnormality might include a normal wave occurring at the wrong time. For example, delta waves that are seen during reading or performing a simple math problem are abnormal and could account for errors. And the appearance of theta waves while in a classroom setting or driving on the highway is abnormal and could account for poor comprehension or "human error."

The ability to produce alpha waves is associated with an overall healthy brain and body, especially in relation to controlling stress. It is one reason people have, for thousands of years, pursued meditation, the use of psychedelics and other drugs, prayer and other activities that seek to promote the alpha state. Specifically, alpha waves can reduce high levels of the stress hormone cortisol, and help balance the autonomic nervous system. These alpha waves can have dramatic effects on the entire body, such as improved memory, learning and comprehension, better blood-sugar regulation, improved gut function, and balanced hormones. When we're relaxed, creative, meditating and happy, the brain produces large amounts of alpha waves.

The *inability* to produce alpha waves is abnormal. Blood sugar problems, inadequate sleep, nutritional imbalance and very high levels of stress hormones can impair the ability to produce alpha waves. Even certain mechanical imbalances, such as those in the jaw joint or neck muscles can significantly reduce the ability to generate healthy alpha waves.

An easy method of promoting alpha wave production is called *respiratory biofeedback*. I developed this procedure, sometimes called the *5-Minute Power Break*, by combining two powerful therapies: the first is manual biofeedback that helps muscles function better (and discussed in Chapter 30), and the second is neurofeedback, or EEG biofeedback, which helps improve brain function.

Respiratory Biofeedback

One of the most powerful brain and body remedies I've ever used is called respiratory biofeedback. You can perform it yourself as a quick, effective daily therapy to reduce stress, relax and improve overall health. Here are some of its significant health benefits:

- It can increase oxygen to the brain, potentially improving a variety of neurological imbalances. This is accomplished through more efficient breathing that brings more air into the lungs.

- It can increase the brain's production of alpha waves. These brain waves can help reduce harmful stress hormones, balance the nervous system and promote relaxation — very important features for a healthier brain and body.

- Respiratory feedback can help restore normal breathing. Improper breathing is often associated with brain and spinal cord injuries, and is sometimes a hidden problem even in relatively healthy people.

- It can improve the function of the diaphragm and abdominal muscles. In addition to breathing, these muscles play a significant role in physical movement, improving posture and supporting the spine and pelvis.

- Because of its effect on the brain and nervous system, respiratory biofeedback can improve the function of other muscles in the body as well, and help reduce pain.

Here are the steps for respiratory biofeedback:

- It's best performed in a lying position, although slightly reclined while sitting is also effective.

- Place the hands or arms on the middle of the abdomen, and keep them relaxed. This provides a biofeedback effect on the diaphragm and abdominal muscles during movement.

- Closing the eyes can increase healthy alpha brain waves.

- Listening to enjoyable music is also a great way to increase alpha waves, especially if headphones are used which keeps out distracting noise.

- Breathe easy. Most people can comfortably, slowly inhale for about five to seven seconds; then, exhale for the same five to seven seconds. If five to seven seconds makes you feel out of breath or dizzy, adjust the time — try three to four seconds during inhalation, for example, and the same for exhalation.

- Continue respiratory biofeedback for about five minutes.

Caution: It's very important to not fall asleep, or not even start drifting into sleep. If this happens, discontinue the respiratory biofeedback session. Sleep produces very different brain waves (delta waves, as noted above) that should be avoided during respiratory biofeedback. If you start getting sleepy after two minutes, perform respiratory biofeedback for just less than that time and gradually work up to five minutes — but always avoid getting sleepy. If you consistently get sleepy during respiratory biofeedback, there may be other sleep-related issues such as sleep deprivation or sleep apnea.

Respiratory biofeedback can be performed once or twice daily, or even more if necessary. Many people feel so much better afterward, and can tell when it's time to perform it. And, before the implementation of other therapies (massage, yoga, chiropractic, etc.), it's best to perform respiratory biofeedback first because it can help make these therapies more successful.

Rest and Stimulation

Two other very important factors for optimal brain function are rest and stimulation. Brain rest comes in the form of sleep. For the average adult, sleeping uninterrupted for at least seven and no more than nine hours is normal; children need more. Some people believe they could function well on less sleep, but they probably can't. And too much sleep may be associated with certain disorders, including depression.

The best environment for a sleeping brain (and body) is in a dark and quiet comfortable clutter-free bedroom. The sensations of light and sound can keep the brain from resting. Creating this environment is usually easy to do.

No other body area responds better than the brain to the notion of "use it or lose it." This comes in the form of mental stimulation. In addition to food and nutrition, exercise and controlling stress, continually using the brain is important. This includes providing it with new information such as a language or touch-typing, or reading interesting information with which you're not familiar. It also means doing physical things your brain is not familiar with such as using your opposite hand for eating, changing physical routines or performing other uncommon tasks. In addition, easy aerobic exercise is one of the most powerful brain therapies because many of the nerves in the muscles begin in the brain — each muscle contraction and relaxation is a unique and healthy brain stimulation.

In addition, one of the best brain therapies is to follow your passion. If that's painting, pottery, climbing a mountain or whatever — pursue it and do it! Included in this is a simple motto: Do the things you're good at doing; avoid things you don't do well (or if you love them, learn to do them well).

And don't forget music — just listening is a powerful way to stimulate the brain. Watching music videos, playing music and writing it are also great workouts for the brain. Music can stimulate more areas of the brain at one time than almost anything else.

Music Matters

Do you want to know a secret? Like food, nutrition and exercise, music can play an eloquent role in improving your quality of life. There's nothing like listening to Mozart, the Beatles or Cat Stevens to reduce stress or meditatively ponder life. There's a place for Chopin, and Dylan. Match the music and your mood, and you're on your way.

Music may not always be a magical mystery tour, but it sure can do something unique. Scientists have shown beneficial effects of music on controlling stress, reducing pain, and improving immune and brain function. Music around mealtime can help digestion, too. After a hard day's night, or if you've been working eight days a week, relaxing and listening to some good music can help. Everything seems to come together, emotionally, in a healthy, therapeutic way.

Music as therapy is thousands of years old. Perhaps the first written therapeutic use came from Chinese medicine about 5,000 years ago. About 2500 BC, followers of Pythagoras developed a science of musical psychotherapy. Today, the long and winding road of music includes treatment for many types of patients, including those with depression, autism, learning disabilities, Alzheimer's and others. But almost anyone can enjoy the music as well as its health benefits.

It's not necessary to know the musical key associated with particular areas of the body, as taught in Chinese medicine, because the particular music that is most therapeutic is the music you like. Most likely, the music you find most comforting includes tunes from yesterday — those associated with good memories, typically from when you were younger. This is the basis for using music in the treatment of brain disorders, from simple memory problems to more serious diseases. Stimulating auditory sense is just one way to trigger emotions with potentially therapeutic outcomes. Another way is visual — watching a music video, or being at a concert may even be more powerful. Applying the kinesthetic sense — the act of playing music, for example — can even be more potent. Add some dancing (you can even twist and shout) and now you've added more brain stimulation with an aerobic complement.

Directed at consumers, music equals money: Studies show that background music can bring increased sales. This subliminal use of music has been used for centuries. And many of the successful radio and TV commercials use well-known music to sell products.

Just as we can use a healthy snack in place of junk food, so too can music rescue us from things like television, unpleasant get-togethers and other unhealthy activities. So pull those old records out of the attic, or buy some new CDs — think of it like you're buying organic vegetables or grass-fed beef. Dig it.

The End.

29

The Gut

The main function of the gastrointestinal tract — the gut — is digestion of food and absorption of nutrients. Most people are well aware of these activities, but the gut is also home to most of the adult immune system. It also assists the liver by eliminating toxins, produces vitamins and hormones, has an extensive nervous system of its own and is in constant communication with the brain. When the gut is under stress, all these areas can be significantly disturbed. For example, even if you eat the right foods, if they're not digested, and if the small intestine does not absorb nutrients, malabsorption can cause nutritional imbalances. This could create a problem identical to those associated with not eating the right foods.

Although a variety of supplements can help remedy intestinal dysfunction and are described in this chapter, it's important to avoid the temptation to use the many products on the market — from dietary supplements to drugs — that claim to fix your gut. That's because getting your whole body healthy with the topics discussed throughout this book can improve intestinal function — often dramatically.

Symptoms of gut dysfunction are another epidemic in today's high-stress, bad food society. Among the biggest sellers of drugs, both over-the-counter and prescriptions, are those that cover the symptoms of an improperly functioning gut. And it should not be a surprise to learn that many of these drugs, prescriptions too, are given to children (despite not being approved for them). But the majority of gut problems can be significantly improved or eliminated by making some relatively easy changes in your food intake and controlling stress. These problems include issues in the mouth, such as cavities and other tooth problems, indigestion, ulcers, reflux and other chronic diseases such as Crohn's and ulcerative colitis. Among the common problems are inflammatory conditions — those names ending in "itis." From the mouth (gingivitis) to the large intestine (colitis), inflammation is the end result of a chronic condition that includes an imbalance of fats as previously discussed. Restoring fat balance is a key step to eliminating inflammatory problems. In addition, ulcers are specifically part of the inflammatory process; treating an ulcer begins with restoring a balance of fats.

The Mouth

We use it for talking, singing, screaming, kissing and even making odd noises. It's the mouth, and it serves another important function that many people neglect — helping us get more nutrients from our food and keep our gut working well. Many gut problems begin in the mouth, and many can be significantly improved by using the mouth more. Gut problems can come from not chewing food, which may be due to problems with the teeth or jaw joint (TMJ), and low salivary pH. Most often, however, it's due to rushing meals, poor eating habits or never having learned to properly chew your food.

Chewing

Russian physiologist Ivan Pavlov's groundbreaking research into the importance of chewing and human digestion won him a Nobel Prize in 1904. After more than a century, physiologists continue building on that understanding of the benefits of chewing.

The taste receptors on the tongue detect extremely small concentrations of substances within a fraction of a second of tasting it — one reason we love the taste of food. This stimulation elicits a variety of immediate responses throughout the body, including stimulating heat production and fat-burning, and improving digestion, absorption and even the use of nutrients from foods. Chewing our food, called the "cephalic phase" of digestion, can also help control blood sugar and control fluid and mineral balance.

Chewing of foods with various tastes, textures and temperatures is an important oral stimulation for everyone, especially for the very young and the elderly. Infants with increased oral stimulation grow better with fewer medical complications, and the elderly benefit with improved digestive function and better overall health. And, exercising the TMJ and other mouth and face muscles keep them fit and improve the vital circulation around teeth and in the gums for optimal oral hygiene.

All food should be chewed. But those that require the most chewing include concentrated carbohydrates — bread and other starchy grain products, including pasta, rice and beans, all cereals, starchy vegetables such as potatoes and corn, and all sugars (the exceptions are fruit and honey which don't require chemical digestion). An important enzyme in saliva starts digestion of these foods, and without it normal digestion of these carbohydrates may not occur, with the risk of producing gas, indigestion and other intestinal problems.

Keep it simple: Rather than counting each mouthful, just chew and enjoy the tastes and textures of the food you're eating. Once it has turned into very small pieces and well moistened, swallow it and enjoy another bite. Rushing meals, eating while working and other poor habits makes it almost impossible to chew and digest well. Listening to music during meals in a relaxed environment can help all phases of digestion.

Oral pH

The environment of the mouth is an important part of its overall health, especially the acid-alkaline balance — the pH — of the saliva. The pH can be measured with pH paper, available at a pharmacy, health store or online. The pH of the mouth should be slightly alkaline, in the range of about 7.2 to 7.6 (slightly higher in children). You may hear or read that the mouth should be an acid pH, but this is confused by the fact that most people have a mouth with a pH in the acid range — 6.0, 6.5, 6.8, etc. (A pH of 7.0 is neutral; above is alkaline and below is acid.)

Here's the procedure to test your pH:

1. Wait at least 15 minutes after eating or drinking.

2. Use a small strip of pH paper and thoroughly moisten it in your mouth for about five to 10 seconds.

3. Immediately compare the color on your test strip with

the color on the pH paper container to determine the approximate pH.

Initially, perform this test two or three times a day, then again a few days later to establish your average pH level, although it should not vary by much. If your pH is consistently too high (above 7.6), it may indicate a need to increase natural carbohydrates such as fruits and whole grains. But if your pH is too low it may indicate two things: You're eating too much carbohydrate and you also need to add more protein and fat to the diet. After making the appropriate dietary changes, check the pH twice a week to follow progress as improvements in pH could take up to a month or more.

In children and adults, low pH — less than 7.0 — promotes tooth decay. While in practice I noticed children (and adults) with proper pH did not get cavities, and those who had tooth decay almost always had low pH. (Low pH may also indicate reduced fat-burning, excess stress or sometimes other nutritional problems.)

The Stomach

Of all the problems associated with the stomach, perhaps most are related to hydrochloric acid. This normal acid is a vital part of the digestive process. Without its action, nutrient availability may be greatly diminished due to poor digestion and malabsorption, and the risk of disease is increased.

These problems are usually due to low levels of hydrochloric acid (hypochlorhydria) or a lack of acid (achlorhydria). Stress, illness and aging are the most common reasons for reduction of natural hydrochloric acid in the stomach. This results in diminished digestion of a variety of nutrients, from calcium and zinc, to iron, vitamin B12 and protein. Problems are not limited to the stomach, but throughout the gut. For example, hydrochloric acid in the stomach stimulates the production of pancreatic and other digestive enzymes in the small intestine — without adequate stomach acid poor small intestine function follows. Another problem associated with low stomach acid is the presence of bacteria, viruses, parasites, yeast or fungus — the stomach should not contain any of these organisms and normal stomach acid is a defense against these organisms. In addition to many types of gut problems, low stomach acid is found in people with other conditions including rheumatoid arthritis, asthma, atherosclerosis and candida yeast infections.

Most problems associated with hydrochloric acid are related to diminished production. However, sometimes an excess of stomach acid is produced. This is one of the rationales for giving antacids. In some people, strong emotional stress can overproduce hydrochloric acid between meals when the stomach is empty. This is not normal and is clearly a health problem. In these cases, the stress must be addressed, and eating more frequently, as often as six times a day, is usually very helpful.

Other acids can also be overproduced in the stomach due to low hydrochloric acid levels. This occurs when food is eaten and the stomach has too little hydrochloric acid. This may be followed by formation of other acids from fermentation and poor digestion, and can result in a condition of "too much acid" — caused by too little normal acid. Antacids can relieve discomfort caused by these unnatural acids, and this has resulted in an explosion of antacid products both in over-the-counter and prescription forms.

Taking antacids may be counterproductive for efficient digestion and absorption, especially when low stomach acid already exists. The drugs used to "neutralize" stomach acids don't really accomplish this. They just temporarily reduce the acids, the reason you have to continue taking the drug. Improving the diet and reducing stress, however, can help remedy this problem in most people. For those who need more help, a dietary supplement can be very effective.

For those who require more stomach acid, betaine hydrochloride is the name of the ingredient in dietary supplements that can increase the normal stomach acid. This is a natural product — it's actually the salt of hydrochloric acid in dry form, which turns into the same stomach acid when swallowed. It's best taken after meals and snacks until intestinal function returns to normal. In some people a long-term need for betaine hydrochloride exists, especially in the elderly. Betaine hydrochloride is typically supplemented at a dose of 100-600 mg after each meal and snack.

Many supplements containing betaine hydrochloride also include digestive enzymes, such as pancreatic and other small intestine enzymes. Because the normal stomach acid stimulates the production of pancreatic enzymes in the small intestine, I prefer to use betaine hydrochloride without additional digestive enzymes in most cases.

Reflux

GERD — gastroesophageal reflux — has become a commonly diagnosed problem in both children and adults. Drugs to treat the symptoms are among the biggest sellers, yet people still have the symptoms. In true cases of GERD, stomach contents back up into the esophagus, causing irritation, with symptoms occurring mostly after meals, or when lying down or bending over with the head below the waist. In severe cases, ulceration can occur in the esophagus. Most people have less serious but sometimes very uncomfortable symptoms associated with bloating due to gas. This often comes from eating starchy or processed carbohydrates, especially at the same time as eating dense proteins, overeating and other causes of gas (see sidebar on gas). Reducing or eliminating carbohydrates, including lactose from dairy, often eliminates the symptoms of GERD. In other cases, poor stomach digestion (not enough stomach acid) causes the symptoms as discussed above.

Don't Water-Down Your Meals

Maintaining a healthy stomach is important during meals. Stress may be the biggest and most common culprit. But drinking water with meals adds another stress to stomach function. People commonly consume a glass or two of water during a meal. This can reduce the stomach's ability to effectively digest its food and increase the amount of air in the stomach, another potential stress that reduces digestion. For many people, drinking water with meals becomes a habit because they do not chew their food well. Proper chewing moistens food sufficiently eliminating the need for additional liquids. Small amounts of wine or other non-sweetened alcohol as a liquid can help digestion, but other than that, liquids should be consumed between, not during meals. Drink water about 15 or 20 minutes *before* meals and about an hour *after* meals.

Be Careful with Food Combinations

Another important consideration for healthy stomach function is the rate of digestion of different foods, the main issue underlying the notion of proper food combining. The worst foods to combine in the stomach at the same time are proteins and carbohydrates. Concentrated protein foods, such as meat, fish, eggs and cheese, digest at much different rates than concentrated carbohydrate foods such as grains, potatoes and most sugars. Since fruit, honey and fiber don't require chemical digestion, they won't interfere with protein foods in the stomach during digestion. Common combinations of foods in our society contribute to the epidemic of gut problems: eggs and toast, a cheese sandwich, spaghetti and meatballs, a sugary dessert after a protein meal, and so many other unhealthy habits.

Instead of these meals, have a vegetable omelet, a salad with cheese, spaghetti squash with meatballs, and fruit or a honey-based dessert. Or, if you're eating a carbohydrate meal such as beans and brown rice, mostly carbohydrates with little protein, combine it with vegetables and avoid the cheese.

When food completes its digestion in the stomach, which may take up to two hours depending on the foods, with high-fat meals taking longer, it enters the small intestine.

The Small Intestine

The digestion of food continues in the small intestine, where most nutrients get absorbed into the bloodstream. In addition to enzymes made in the small intestine, pancreatic enzymes and bile from the gall bladder are added to the food to help in the process. Poor digestion in the stomach usually produces poor digestion in the small intestine. And poor digestion results in poor absorption of nutrients called malabsorption.

Malabsorption is not an uncommon problem stemming from stress, antibiotic use, poor stomach function or other causes. The diminished ability of the small intestine to absorb nutrients, from calcium and zinc to vitamin B12, iron and protein, leads to numerous health issues.

Many patients who consulted me through the years showed a need for additional nutrients. While it was tempting to urge my patients to take all these nutrients in supplement form, the problem was often not the lack of nutrients but the inability of the body to absorb them. In fact, some patients showed the need for certain nutrients they had been taking in supplement form for months or even years! Improving stomach and intestinal function, including absorption, eliminated the need for most of these supplemental nutrients because the patient could now obtain them from food.

An effective dietary supplement to help protect against and remedy the common problem of malabsorption is the amino acid L-glutamine. This nutrient is the primary energy source for the villi of the small intestine — the structures that actually absorb nutrients from food. These delicate villi are easily damaged or destroyed under stress, by poor eating habits, by fasting or illness, and glutamine helps restore their function. Glutamine also reduces intestinal distress, improves immunity, has an anti-inflammatory effect, and can protect the intestines from the dangers of aspirin and other harmful chemicals.

Glutamine is available in powder form or capsules. But if you add glutamine to liquids, be sure to consume it right away; if it remains in liquid it begins to lose potency. Most people don't need to take glutamine for long periods. Once the gut is healed and working well it should be discontinued. About 500 to 1,000 mg once or twice daily is a common dose. The need for glutamine is another example of a high-dose supplement that can be valuable in some individuals.

Liver Detox

The liver plays an important role in intestinal function. One of the most important of the liver's thousands of jobs is disarming toxins by chemically breaking them down and removing them through the intestine — via bile through the gall bladder.

By filtering the blood, the liver breaks down and eliminates an untold number of toxins that are produced within the body during normal metabolism, and those that enter the body through food and the environment. This is accomplished through a complex process referred to as *detoxification*, which requires a variety of nutrients that must come from the diet. Many scams lure the public with their miracle liver detox potions, but the very best way to promote healthy liver function comes from eating real food and avoiding environmental toxins as much as possible.

Of the many nutrients required for liver detox, how do we know which are needed most? The answer is they're all important — with many more valuable nutrients in foods yet to be discovered. So a diet full of a variety of organic, unprocessed foods — fresh vegetables and fruits, whole nuts and seeds, and high-quality protein (including whole eggs) — should contain adequate amounts to support liver detox. Organic foods have more of these important nutrients and fewer toxins such as pesticides (an additional burden for the liver).

The signs and symptoms of poor liver detox may be very subtle. So how do you know if your liver function needs more support? Ask yourself the following questions:

❏ Are you sensitive to caffeine (can consume only small amounts or none at all)?

❏ Are you sensitive to perfumes, paints and other chemical smells?

❏ Are you sensitive to certain drugs: benzodiazepines (Valium, Ativan, Xanax), antihistimines (Benadryl, Claritin), certain antibiotics (Bactrim, Erythromycin) and antifungals (Lotrimin)?

❏ Are you sensitive to certain foods: grapefruit, turmeric, curry, chili (capsaicin) or cloves?

❏ Do you eat less than two servings a day of animal protein (meat, fish, whole eggs)?

❏ Are you taking non-steroidal anti-inflammatory drugs (Advil, Aleve)?

❏ Are you taking more than one dose of Tylenol or aspirin per week?

❏ Are you sensitive (even to the smell) to high sulfur-containing foods such as egg yolks, onions, garlic, broccoli or cabbage?

❏ Do you consume more than two alcoholic drinks per day?

❏ Do you eat less than about eight serving of vegetables and fruits per day?

If you answered "yes" to even one or two of these questions, it could indicate poor liver detoxification. Liver function also slows down with age if you don't keep it going with adequate healthy food.

Note: For ease of study, biochemists discuss liver detox as two chemical pathways, called Phase I and Phase II. Each is associated with specific toxins and nutrients. For simplicity, we're grouping them together as "liver detox." It is important to understand that too much of one nutrient, even as a food dose, may help one phase while hurting the other. Balance and moderation are key.

Glutathione: The Detox Key

The single most important compound for liver detox is a substance called glutathione, the most powerful of antioxidants that the body produces. No single food is high in this natural substance, nor can we take it in supplement form because it's unstable. Fortunately, the body makes glutathione when we eat a variety of foods and food-based supplements rich in specific nutrients. Some of the key nutrients the body needs to make glutathione include:

- Lipoic acid found in spinach, broccoli, peas, Brussels sprouts and many other bitter vegetables.

- Sulforaphan from broccoli and kale (highest in broccoli sprouts).

- Gamma tocopherol and alpha tocotrienol from fresh vegetables, nuts and seeds.

- The amino acid cysteine, highest in certain animal proteins, especially whey.

Free Radical Fallout

The process of detoxification normally produces large amounts of unstable chemicals called oxygen free radicals. A diet rich in *antioxidants* helps sweep up this radical "fall-out" of liver detox. Potent antioxidants found in brightly colored vegetables and fruits include the carotenoids (lycopene, beta carotene, zeaxanthin, lutein) and the full vitamin E complex, especially beta, delta and gamma tocopherol. Food doses of vitamin C (found in the whites of red peppers and citrus, and many other fruits and vegetables) also work with other antioxidants.

To spice up your healthy meals, include foods rich in phytonutrients that also assist liver detox. These include citrus peel (make a citrus peel zest, or a marmalade with honey), caraway seeds (grind them just before use), turmeric, ginger, garlic and dill, just to name a few.

Liver detoxification also requires B vitamins, especially thiamine (B1), niacin (B3) and the folates. But avoid the synthetic forms because these have to be *detoxed* and eliminated through the liver too. Alcohol, in small amounts, can actually help liver detox. In moderation, alcohol is broken down in the liver but by a different mechanism that also requires B vitamins. But excessive alcohol taps into Phase II detoxification where it can cause significant stress.

Other Liver Stresses

If you have a history of liver problems, there are certain foods and drugs best avoided. These include iron from dietary supplements, alcohol and products containing acetaminophen (including Tylenol, Excedrin and other aspirin-free products). These substances can add significant chemical stress to the liver. In addition, avoid the foods you're sensitive to, and be especially aware of caffeine; if you don't tolerate it, avoid it!

The liver eliminates toxins through the gall bladder and transports them into the intestines with the help of bile. Fatty foods keep bile flowing, helping the liver do this job. Very low fat diets can reduce bile production and can be dangerous. Likewise, very high fat diets can overwork the gall bladder.

Improving liver function is a key to helping the entire intestine function in a normal healthy way, especially the large intestine.

Large Intestine

The colon, or large intestine, also plays a significant role in overall health. Problems can arise within the colon, or because the foods passing into it have not been properly digested. For example, low lev-

Food Intolerance

I've discussed carbohydrate intolerance in great detail, but various other foods can also cause problems generally labeled as food intolerance. Symptoms come from various reactions in the body, although the gut is usually the main area of involvement. Intestinal gas, nausea, diarrhea and abdominal discomfort are the most common indications. More serious food intolerances can cause skin reactions, such as a rash or welts, breathing difficulties, such as wheezing and asthma symptoms, head and sinus problems including inflammation, runny eyes and nose, and headache, and whole body reactions such as edema (fluid retention) or even shock.

In addition to carbohydrates, including lactose (milk sugar), fructose and the so-called "sugar-free" sugars sorbitol, mannitol and xylitol, other foods can sometimes cause bad reactions. These include:

- Monosodium glutamate (MSG), commonly used in packed foods and in restaurants;

- Sulfites, which naturally occur in red wine, but are sometimes sprayed on vegetables and fruits (another reason to eat organic).

- Histamine-containing foods, including beer, wine, cheese, chocolate, tomatoes, saurkraut, vinegar, eggplant, spinach, some fish (tuna and mackerel) and yeast.

- A variety of additives and other agents used to make dietary supplements, medications, and cosmetics can also trigger reactions.

els of hydrochloric acid can cause stress in the colon from undigested food. This can cause irritation directly, or influence the "friendly" bacteria that should be living there.

While most of the gut — from stomach through the small intestine — is sterile, the large intestine is home to various types of bacteria that normally reside there. They help create an important environ-

Intestinal Gas

When too much gas accumulates in the intestine, it can cause more than discomfort. Pockets of gas anywhere in the gut can trigger a sympathetic nervous system response — a stress reaction. Small amounts of gas in the gut are normal. But larger volumes of gas are not normal, usually indicating something is wrong with your diet or even the way you're eating. Here are the four most common causes of intestinal gas:

- The most common cause is starchy carbohydrates — bread, cereal, the many products made from wheat flour — and sugar and sugar-containing foods. This includes milk sugar (lactose) from dairy products. Review the carbohydrate chapters if you're not sure which carbohydrates can adversely affect digestion and health.

- Another common cause of intestinal gas is swallowing air. This occurs during eating and drinking liquids, especially water, as people tend to drink several ounces or more at one time. Drink liquids slowly to avoid swallowing air, and most importantly keep your head level — not tilted backward — to avoid swallowing air. In addition, chewing food and not rushing meals will help you avoid swallowing large amounts of air. Once air is swallowed, if it doesn't come back up

ment for making nutrients, including biotin, some of the B vitamins and vitamin K, and for generating energy. Many strains of bacteria have been used for centuries as cultured foods such as yogurt and kefir, and in more recent times dietary supplements containing freeze-dried forms. These bacteria strains include lactobacillus (containing acidophilus, rhamnosus and salivarius), bifidobacterium bifidum and streptococcus thermophilus. Supplements containing these types of bacteria are called "probiotics." (Prebiotic foods, which help feed these bacterial, were discussed in a previous chapter.)

soon as a burp, most of it must travel through the gut and come out the other end.

- Stomach dysfunction is a common cause of gas. This is typically due to low levels of hydrochloric acid as discussed above.

- Large intestine dysfunction — often due to the wrong bacteria residing in the gut (also discussed above) may cause excess gas. This can also cause bad breath as some of this gas is absorbed into the blood and released through the lungs.

- Combinations of these problems also may result in significant gas in the gut.

Other foods that promote gas include chewing gum, especially the "sugar-free" products containing sorbitol and other alcohol sugars. In addition, some individuals are sensitive to the natural fruit sugar fructose found in fruits, and especially high in fruit juice.

Drugs to reduce gas don't work. The American College of Gastroenterology states, "Despite the many commercials and advertisements for medications which reduce gas pains and bloating, very few have any proven scientific value." If you have excess gas, addressing the causes as discussed here can usually significantly reduce the problem.

The most common indication for the need of a probiotic supplement is when the friendly bacteria are replaced by other unhealthy bacteria. This occurs with antibiotic use. Stress associated with travel, and excess stress in general, poor diet and other problems also contribute to poor intestinal function associated with the need for probiotics. Signs and symptoms associated with poor intestinal bacteria include diarrhea and constipation, foul-smelling gas and stool, indigestion and many of the common illnesses such as irritable bowel syndrome, colitis and ileitis, and others.

In seeking the best probiotic products, consider these factors:

- Read the label for the numbers of each bacteria strain per serving (not per bottle). These should be listed in billions, not millions.

- Be sure there are enough varieties of bacteria, especially the ones noted above.

- Check the expiration date as even freeze-dried bacteria eventually die.

- Bacterial cultures that last the longest are those that are kept refrigerated.

- A healthy diet helps these supplemental bacteria maintain the friendly bacteria in the intestine, especially the "prebiotics" food as previously discussed.

The gut also has many far-reaching influences throughout the body. The gut is the home of much of an adult's immune system, and the health of the overall body is influenced by the intestine. The potential for allergy is gut-related as absorption of undigested proteins can trigger allergic reaction, which can affect the skin, sinuses, immune system and even the gut itself. Food intolerances, previously discussed, are also gut-related. And in recent years, the idea of a "gut-brain" connection has begun to develop, with significant influence on the brain from the gut's overall health.

How do you know when the gut is working best? The answer seems obvious but it's a common question. Most people don't feel different after taking a probiotic supplement, for example, or implementing other seeming healthy habits for the gut. Clearly, you should not just feel better, but function better when the proper combinations of food changes, dietary supplements and other lifestyle factors are implemented. You should not have indigestion or large amounts of gas. You should have one, two or three bowel movements per day that are not foul-smelling. In addition, if you start taking a probiotic supplement, or otherwise improve gut bacteria (such as with yogurt or other cultured foods), the result should be a noticeable increase in stool bulk. Consider that almost half of the stool may be bacteria.

With the wrong bacteria residing in the gut, stool content may be low. But with the proper bacteria in the large intestine, stool bulk can increase by as much as 45 percent.

Case History

CR was diagnosed with ulcerative colitis more than 10 years before coming to my clinic. This chronic inflammatory condition, including significant losses of blood, frequent diarrhea and extreme fatigue not only was a serious health problem but it was wrecking her entire life. The medications that were keeping CR alive had many side effects, and each year, on one or two occasions, she would get so ill that hospitalization was the only option. She resisted surgery, and as a last resort was willing to try a more natural approach one more time.

After extensive evaluations, I recommended that CR strictly adhere to a healthy lifestyle to quickly pull her out of the viscous cycle she was in for most of her adult life. She made significant dietary changes beginning with the Two-Week Test. It was evident that CR had to eliminate all grains and starchy carbohydrates, eat smaller more frequent meals, and eliminate all processed and packaged foods. She started taking a number of supplements, including fish oil, L-glutamine, betaine hydrochloride, a natural form of folic acid, and probiotics. She listened to the music she loved whenever possible during the day, and made a great effort to avoid the people and activities in her life that caused her stress.

Within a couple of weeks, CR was noticeably improved, and after a month her intestinal function was significantly better. After another month she quickly weaned off all medication. By six months she claimed there were no symptoms of colitis — no discomfort, no bleeding and normal bowel movements. A visit to her gastroenterologist showed significant healing of her colon, and blood tests were dramatically improved. CR continued to see me about twice a year without return of any problems, except on occasion when she would eat improperly during travel or holidays — but eventually she was able to resolve these problems too.

Acid-Alkaline Balance

Nutritionally, a healthy diet does more than provide nutrients. Through digestion of these foods, an important biochemical acid-alkaline balance occurs, which significantly helps maintain overall health. The kidneys play a vital role in this pH balance too.

There are many hyped-up products and diets in the marketplace claiming to save us from dietary acidosis by making the body alkaline. Certainly an imbalance in our acid-alkaline state can seriously disrupt your health, but simply balancing the foods consumed accomplishes this better than any so-called "miracle product" (at 10 times the cost of real food), and this addresses the cause of the problem rather than taking a supplement to treat symptoms.

For almost all of human existence a slightly alkaline diet has been the norm. This is considered to be optimal. With the agricultural revolution of the past five to 10 thousand years came a dramatic rise in processed grain consumption, which significantly added more acid-producing foods to the diet, disturbing the balance. Grain foods also replaced many vegetables and fruits in the diet, which were primarily those needed to maintain a healthy alkaline state. Today, most "Westernized" diets are full of highly processed grains, especially wheat, contributing to an over-acid state. Excessive animal protein intake can also make the body more acidic.

Most foods produce either an acid or alkaline residue. This affects the whole body via the bloodstream. Foods that are most acid-producing include grains (both whole and processed), milk products, meat, fish, eggs and salt. Foods most alkaline include vegetables, fruits and nuts. Fats and legumes are neutral. If we eat too much acid or too much alkaline food, we risk creating an imbalance. For most people, the risk comes from eating too much acid food. Typically this is from too many grains such as bread and cereal, but too much milk and meat also contribute. When the body becomes too acid, many problems can arise. Because the kidneys must work hard to re-establish the acid-alkaline balance, they can become overworked, especially if water intake is not sufficient. Eating too many acid-producing foods can result in a general bodywide imbalance — a state of chronic acidosis. This can cause bone and muscle problems, such as fractures, osteoporosis, muscle weakness and muscle wasting. With aging, this increases the risk of falls, fractures and disability, and also leads to the loss of independence, all of which contributes to increased mortality and reduced quality of life. Many other problems can develop too, such as kidney disease, high blood pressure, poor mineral balance (with significant loss of magnesium), asthma, cardiovascular disease and other conditions.

The answer to the problem of acid-alkaline imbalance is not to create an opposite imbalance by over-consuming a high alkaline product or eliminating all acid foods. Such is the case, for example, when high-quality animal protein is eliminated from the diet (which can actually worsen bone and muscle problems). Rather, establishing balance in the diet is a key to an optimal acid-alkaline state. It means eating sufficiently from both the healthy acid and alkaline food groups. For most people, this means eating more fresh vegetables and fruits; 10 servings a day for adults, and proportional amounts for children based on body weight. It may also mean eliminating refined grain products.

All areas of the gastrointestinal tract — the gut — are vital for optimal health and human performance. Any area not functioning well needs attention. Improving gut function not only can help the intestine work better, but you'll absorb more nutrients from foods, and the whole body and brain will work better.

Constipation and Diarrhea

Constipation and diarrhea are among the most common gut complaints. Most people can avoid or resolve these problems by being fit and healthy. Constipation technically refers to excess straining with bowel movements and the passage of small hard stools. It can occur when the waste (stool) moves too slowly through the lower gut. The most common causes include dehydration, changes in diet (this may occur initially, even when improving your diet), physical inactivity and a variety of drugs. Treatment and prevention includes drinking sufficient water between meals, 10 servings of vegetables & fruits (prunes are very effective — one to three per day with a large glass of water), psyllium taken with a large glass of water and physical activity such as regular walking. In almost all cases, these habits will result in normal gut function (having at least one to three bowel movements a day). However, if more remedies are needed to treat constipation, it's best to see your doctor.

Diarrhea is an abnormal looseness of the stools, usually with increased frequency. Acute watery diarrhea, with symptoms of gas, cramping and intestinal pain, is usually associated with some illness . When severe it can lead to dehydration and dangerous losses of electrolytes (including sodium, potassium, calcium and magnesium). Acute diarrhea is often caused by a viral infection, and sometimes by drugs, especially antibiotics. Bacterial infections are sometimes the cause, especially when blood is present. Artificial sweeteners, especially the alcohol sugars sorbitol, xylitol and others, can also cause acute diarrhea. If you have acute diarrhea lasting more than 10 days or two weeks see your doctor. When acute diarrhea becomes chronic it may be associated with more serious problems. NSAIDS, antibiotics and antacids can also cause chronic diarrhea, as can dairy foods and gluten-containing grains — especially wheat. Finding and eliminating the cause of the problem is the best remedy. In the meantime, keeping well hydrated is important, and pectin, best consumed from fresh apples or applesauce, can be effective as well. The use of pre- and probiotics, as discussed earlier, can also be helpful.

30

Mechanical Fitness and Health

It seems like almost everyone you meet has some type of physical problem with a muscle or joint. Mechanical pain, discomfort and disabilities affect many in the modern world. Back and neck problems, shoulder and wrist pain, chronic hip and knee dysfunction, and other muscle and joint problems are part of the long list of popular complaints.

As common as these conditions are, most are preventable and relatively easy to remedy by improving fitness and health. For example, through the implementation of proper food and nutrition, inflammation can be better controlled (helping to heal and repair physical problems), and building the aerobic system improves muscle function and support of joints and bones. The result often is that many mechanical problems will disappear because the body will correct them. Some get better very quickly, while others may require more time as the body needs to make significant changes in its chemistry and physical structure. Of the remaining mechanical problems, most can be remedied by conservative means, often with the help of the appropriate health-care professional.

This chapter highlights some of the issues related to the common problem of mechanical imbalance. The vast majority of these problems are not permanent. In fact, in addition to allowing the body to correct many of these problems, some can be remedied at home with some simple guidelines. From head and neck, to shoulder, elbow and wrist problems, and down the spine to the hips, knees and feet, most problems are associated with muscle imbalance. This comes from overuse, trauma, or other imbalance caused by brain, spinal or local injury. And, in most chronic situations, muscle imbalance also has a chemical relationship — there is usually an inflammatory factor in the joint, muscle or other area that's part of the problem. Correcting this part of the problem was discussed in relation to balancing fats to control inflammation.

Muscle Imbalance

The combination of muscle weakness and tightness is called muscle imbalance. The most common cause of muscle imbalance is muscle weakness. When this occurs, another muscle or muscles become tight. This pattern of weak and tight can occur anywhere in muscles throughout the body, on the front and back of the arm, thigh, leg, foot or other areas. The result is reduced movement in joints and reduced strength, often leading to pain and disability.

For a better perspective, let me explain about normal muscle movements. In the course of normal activity, muscles become tight as they contract, and looser when relaxed. We can easily feel this in our own muscles. While sitting, place one of your hands under your thigh, with your elbow bent. Then, pull up with your hand, and maintain that contraction. With the fingers of your other hand feel the muscle on the front of your arm, the biceps, and feel how tight it is. Now feel the back of the arm, the triceps muscle, and feel how loose it is. This is a normal pattern of muscle function during most movements.

When there is an imbalance, muscles become abnormally weak (too loose) and too tight; and they feel somewhat similar to the ones in the example above. This state of weakness and tightness can remain for weeks, months or years following some injury. The original injury that first causes muscle weakness can be from a fall, trauma directly to the muscle, overstretching or overuse. But in many cases the cause of the original weakness is well hidden and people don't recall any event that would have caused a problem. And, the severity of the original injury is often not related to level of disability. I've seen severe low back pain that was debilitating — the patient was unable to move much, couldn't get out of bed and was in constant severe pain. But the cause was due to a muscle imbalance that was easily corrected, and the patient did not recall any event and I could not find what caused the problem. (In this case, the patient recovered quickly once the imbalance was corrected and the problem never returned.)

It should be noted that muscles attach to bones through tendons. So when a muscle is not functioning properly, the tendons don't either. Most tendon problems are secondary to muscle imbalance. Likewise, ligaments connect bones to other bones. And, muscles have an important support relationship with both ligaments and bones, directly and indirectly. So when a ligament or bone problem exists, there is usually an associated muscle imbalance.

The cause of muscle imbalance must be addressed if normal muscle balance is to be restored. Sometimes the body can accomplish this, especially when it's fit and healthy overall. In fact, we are always correcting problems because normal wear and tear frequently produces relatively minor imbalances not only in the muscles, but throughout the body. Even without knowing it, the body is always working to restore balance. During the process of correcting its own problems, the body may show relatively minor symptoms, but often none at all. When your body can't fix a particular problem, symptoms develop and you may need additional help. Manual biofeedback is a technique used to help balance muscles.

Manual Biofeedback

Over the past 30-plus years I've developed various biofeedback procedures to help people improve physical balance, reduce stress, increase fat-burning and achieve other benefits. Manual biofeedback is one of these procedures. It encompasses most of the hands-on therapies I've employed and taught to health professionals and lay people throughout my career. Manual biofeedback can help improve muscle imbalance by evaluating and correcting muscle weakness whether from local muscle problems, or brain or spinal cord injury. It's a safe and effective, and relatively easy, approach for use by many individuals, usually producing a rapid response. Manual biofeedback is very useful for almost everyone, including those with common aches and pains and patients with more serious physical ailments, special-needs children and disabled adults.

Most people with mechanical problems fall into at least one of three categories:

- *Local muscle injury* is the most common cause of physical problems, and is often associated with trauma to the muscle itself, such as the result of a fall, a so-called pulled muscle, a twisted ankle or other injury. Micro-trauma is even more common; it's the accumulation of minor physical stress in a muscle or joint, often unnoticed while it's happening, eventually causing a more obvious muscle problem. Too much sitting, repetitive motion and walking in poor-fitting shoes are common examples of micro-trauma that can ultimately cause muscle problems. Local muscle injuries can result in anything from minor annoying achiness to serious or chronic debilitating condition.

- *Brain injury* can occur at any age, even before birth. Trauma, reduced oxygen or nutrient supply, and infections can easily cause brain damage resulting in poor muscle function. A stroke is a common form of brain injury; others include cerebral palsy, Down syndrome and Parkinson's disease. Some brain injuries produce only relatively minor physical problems, such as being uncoordinated or "clumsy."

- An incomplete *spinal cord injury* is often due to physical trauma such as from a serious head or back injury, but a tumor or infection can also be a cause. A spinal cord injury can adversely affect nerves that go to muscles reducing their function. Like a brain injury, spinal cord injuries can cause a wide range of problems, from relatively minor physical ones, to very serious disabilities.

Not long ago, it was assumed that once injured, the brain and spinal cord could not recover. As a result, many of these muscle problems were not successfully treated. But over the last 30 years we've learned that the brain and body, at any age, has an incredible ability to repair itself, even in cases of severe damage. The goal of manual biofeedback is to help the brain and body recover from injury.

Manual biofeedback can help promote and restore muscle balance, and in doing so help improve overall physical movement. Increased movement is a powerful therapy in itself as I previously discussed in relation to the aerobic muscle fibers. Improved movement not only helps locomotion, posture, independence and other areas of fitness, but can also help improve most other areas of the body and brain, including speech, vision, balance, memory and even intellect. And because muscles have other important functions, such as energy production, circulation and immune activity, increasing physical movement can improve overall health.

Manual biofeedback utilizes procedures very similar to standard manual muscle testing — they are part of both the assessment and treatment aspect. Muscle testing is a commonly employed procedure first introduced in 1949 to evaluate muscle weakness in polio patients. Since then, many forms of muscle testing methods have evolved, for both evaluation purposes and treatments. Manual biofeedback incorporates the best of these into one system.

While traditional EMG (electromyography) biofeedback uses computer equipment, including mechanical sensors and electrodes attached to the skin, manual biofeedback does not use any equipment. Instead, manual biofeedback uses another person's neurological sense to convey information and help the patient's brain and body work better. This is a more personalized approach, recruiting more brain-body stimulation with verbal, visual, tactile and other sensory cues that further enlist the patient's participation and motivation. (Much more information on manual biofeedback is available from my website: www.philmaffetone.com.)

Fix Thyself

The concept that the body can fix itself is centuries old. As noted, the first step is to improve overall fitness and health so the body can perform its normal job of correcting imbalances. While many problems can get in the way, two body areas that often interfere with its ability to fix itself are the feet and breathing.

The feet are our physical foundation, and if they are unstable every structure above can become unbalanced, especially the muscles and joints. I discussed two important issues about the feet: the first was finding the best shoes to wear and the second is going barefoot. Both are associated with improving muscle function in the foot, ankle and leg to help maintain a stable foundation. In other words, you'll strengthen chronically weak muscles which will allow tight muscles to relax and restore muscle balance.

Breathing Mechanics

We take breathing for granted, until we have a breathing difficulty. But many people breathe improperly and don't even realize it. Normal breathing is associated with proper muscle movement — the most important being the abdominal muscles in the front and sides of the abdomen, and the diaphragm muscle, which is on top of the abdomen and under the lungs. These muscles move together allowing us to efficiently breathe in and out. With improper breathing, the abdominal and diaphragm muscles work improperly, and many other muscles may not work as well either. In addition, body movement is impaired, oxygen can be reduced and many other problems can occur.

Let's look at the two components of normal breathing, inhalation and exhalation:

- During inhalation the abdominal muscles relax and extend outward, while the diaphragm muscle contracts and moves downward. This allows air to enter the lungs more easily, and is accompanied by a slight whole-body backward extension, especially the spine.

- During exhalation the abdominal muscles contract and tighten, and are gently pulled inward; the diaphragm muscle relaxes with an upward movement. This helps push air out of the lungs, with a slight whole-body flexion.

We can observe or feel another person's breathing and often tell if it's correct, especially watching the belly or feeling it move out on inhalation and in on exhalation. We can also evaluate our own breathing by feeling muscles move:

- Place the palm of one or two of your hands on the abdomen — in the area of your belly button.

- Slowly breathe in and feel the abdominal muscles expand outward. The belly should get bigger during inhalation.

- Now exhale, and feel the abdominal muscles tighten and be pulled inward. The belly is more flat on exhalation.

This is normal breathing. Most movement occurs in the abdominal areas with only slight movement of the chest, which expands more with much deeper breathing.

Those who breathe improperly often move their muscles opposite that of normal. This happens for various reasons. Brain, spinal cord and local muscle injuries can disturb normal movement of the breathing muscles. In some individuals, poor breathing can come from stress, the stigma of not showing a big belly, and even over-exercising the abdominal muscles, making them too tight to relax.

Improving the breathing mechanism can help many areas, including movements of the spine and pelvis, getting more oxygen and eliminating carbon dioxide, and reducing or even eliminating pain.

Pain is an Emotion

There's nothing that interferes with life more than pain. It changes people, their lives and society itself. Pain is often the symptom associated with muscle imbalance, but other causes, such as gut pain are common. Pain medications, which only treat the symptoms not the cause, are among the best selling prescription and over-the-counter drugs.

Pain is an emotion. It originates in nerve endings found in the skin, blood vessels, nerve fibers, joints and bone coverings. Pain nerve endings send messages to the part of the brain responsible for emotions (called the limbic system), where you interpret the feeling as pain. This is why pain is relatively subjective, and an emotion as opposed to a sense, such as the sense of smell, taste, vision or hearing. If pain was a sense, it would be much more difficult, if not practically impossible, to control it by physical (e.g., cold), chemical (e.g., aspirin), or mental (e.g., hypnosis) measures.

The cause of the pain is often in the same physical areas as the pain itself, but at times may be associated with problems elsewhere in the body, or with problems that don't produce symptoms. *Referred pain*, for example, is felt in one location on the body while the cause is somewhere else. A common referred-pain pattern is associated with a heart attack, where pain is felt in the lower neck, shoulder and arm usually on the left side. Or, pain in the middle of the spine may come from an irritation in the stomach. Differentiating the two is sometimes difficult. Referred pain occurs because signals from the stomach and those from the skin (the referred-pain area) "cross" in the spinal cord and when the message gets to the brain it's impossible to differentiate between the origins of the signals.

A mechanical problem in the foot, for example, may not produce pain or other symptoms in the foot itself. But because many foot problems cause instability in the areas above, it may cause pain to occur in the knee. More than half the patient's I've seen with knee pain didn't have primary problems in the knee, but in an asymptomatic foot.

One benefit of pain is that it informs us there's a problem. By doing so, it can help the body compensate (by shifting weight-bearing), and can prevent us from continuing activities that should be avoided. Pain patterns can also help health-care professionals find the cause of a hidden problem.

Pain comes in different forms, depending on its location. For example:

- Mechanical pain can be associated with physical pressure, such as swelling. This type of pain is often described as "stabbing" or "knife-like." Or if associated with blood vessels as "throbbing" or "pounding."

- Chemical pain often comes from inflammation and muscle fatigue. This type of pain is often described as "burning" or "hot."

- Thermal pain from cold or hot temperatures can also produce pain.

And, pain can come from more than one source. Muscle pain, for example, may be from a physical stress, such as swelling, and chemical stress of inflammation. Sunburn pain can come from three types: thermal stress, physical damage to skin and chemical inflammation.

Pain and NSAIDs

Nonsteroidal anti-inflammatory drugs (NSAIDs), including aspirin, ibuprofen (such as Advil) and naproxen (such as Aleve), are commonly used for pain relief. An important observation to make is that if you have pain that improves by taking NSAIDs, it probably indicates you have a fat imbalance as previously discussed.

NSAID side effects often come with many potential problems. These include intestinal bleeding, delayed healing, including bone and cartilage, interference of fat balance, muscle dysfunction, liver and kidney damage, headaches, skin rash, tinnitis (ringing in ears), drowsiness and poor sleep (suppression of melatonin).

Some people continue taking aspirin for pain despite the fact that they do not obtain significant relief or no longer need it. One study showed that 20 of 44 patients who had osteoarthritis were able to stop their regular NSAIDs without return of significant pain, and without other therapy.

Other Muscle Pains

In addition to pain caused by muscle imbalance, other types of muscle pain are common. There are three general types of pain associated with muscles: 1.) Pain experienced during or immediately after physical activity; 2.) Delayed-onset muscle soreness; and 3.) Pain induced by muscle cramps:

- Pain experienced during or immediately after activity usually has a chemical origin. Lactic acid does not cause pain directly, but may be responsible for pH changes associated with pain. Reduced blood flow may also be linked to this type of muscle pain, which will subside quickly once activity is stopped.

- Delayed-onset muscle soreness usually develops within 24 to 48 hours after activity, with a peak in discomfort between 48 and 72 hours. This pain is usually associated with muscle damage. Diminished ranges of motion accompany pain (although muscle dysfunction often continues after pain has resolved).

- Muscle cramps may be due to some type of muscle imbalance, and the reason for the imbalance must be addressed. Proper hydration and the use of sodium or magnesium may be helpful in correcting and preventing muscle cramps, and rarely is potassium or calcium needed. Proper breathing can help prevent and treat diaphragm problems associated with the common "side stitch" type spasms.

Pain Remedies

Prevention of pain is best accomplished by avoiding the stresses that cause it. Over-working, overtraining or otherwise abusing the body typically causes pain. Invariably, many people develop pain, especially related to muscle activity. Here are some factors to consider:

- Home treatment of pain associated with physical activity is best accomplished with cold stimulation — soaking the body area(s) in cold water for 10-15 minutes can be miraculous. Ice is not always needed as cold tap water works great and sometimes ice can cause excessive irritation due to freezing the skin. Use the cold stimulation two or three times the first day, once or twice the second. In most cases, pain is significantly improved quickly.

- The use of heat for pain is a common remedy. However, it can do more harm than good. Inflammation can be worsened with the application of heat. Unless you're quite sure an area is not inflamed, avoid using heat. Most areas of pain, including the joints associated with muscle imbalance, are accompanied by some degree of inflammation.

- Inflammatory pain occurs when fat imbalance produces more pain chemicals — balancing dietary fats (discussed elsewhere) helps prevent chronic inflammation.

- Low-fat diets can worsen pain and increase the risk of other muscular injury.

- The use of NSAIDs should not be a casual thing. Try to avoid any drugs unless absolutely necessary. However, the stress associated with pain may be worse than the drug; in this case the smallest dose for the shortest period of time necessary may be best.

- Many people use alcohol when pain is present, but it can just as easily amplify pain. The pain-reducing ability of alcohol occurs with high doses, something that also creates fat imbalance ultimately increasing pain.

- Simple rubbing of the skin — tactile stimulation — can also control pain. This is accomplished by lightly stroking the skin at or near an area of pain. If you bump your head, you probably subconsciously rub the area. This stimulates large nerve endings in the skin that can block pain sensation in the brain (the same mechanism as electrical nerve stimulation devices).

Pain can be a serious issue, but its cause must be found and eliminated. It may be important to seek professional help to rule out more serious conditions and find the cause. Most pain is due to some mechanical problem and associated with inflammation; these often arise from muscle imbalance. Mechanical problems can often be remedied by improving overall fitness and health.

31

Simplifying Stress

Stress is such an incredibly powerful influence that even if you are doing everything right in terms of diet, nutrition and exercise, it can still crush your efforts to stay healthy. Prolonged periods of too much stress can contribute significantly and directly to many conditions, ranging from reduced quality of life to deadly diseases such as cancer, heart disease, Alzheimer's and many others.

Stress contributes to fatigue, bacterial and viral infections, inflammatory illness, blood-sugar problems, weight gain, intestinal distress, headaches and most other disorders. Stress-related problems account for more than 75 percent of all visits to primary-care physicians and are responsible each day for millions of people needing to take time off work and school. So stress comes with a monetary price tag as well as a toll on your health.

Charles Darwin said it's not the fittest who survive, nor the most intelligent, but those who can best adapt to their environment. Today, we refer to this adaptation as coping.

It's important to remember that stress is a normal part of life and health, and excess stress is not without a remedy. The body has a great coping mechanism for stress — the hormones of the adrenal glands and related nervous system function. However, when the adrenal glands are overworked, bodywide problems can result.

Before discussing the adrenal glands and how we can help protect ourselves from stress, I want to describe what stress is. To simplify stress, I will address the three main types: physical, chemical and mental/emotional. These types of stress can have many different effects. Moreover, each individual responds differently to various combinations of types of stress.

Physical Stress

Physical stresses are strains on the mechanical body. Overworking your muscles is an example of a physical stress. Slight physical stress is what makes exercise beneficial, and is an example of how some stress can help promote health. However, too much physical stress without adequate recovery can potentially result in many problems. Another physical stress is wearing shoes that don't fit right; while you don't always feel it in your feet, it may cause problems elsewhere in your body. Likewise, dental stress can affect more than your mouth, often causing stomach dysfunction, shoulder, neck or head pain. Other physical stresses include poor posture, eye strain and many other situations that adversely impact the mechanical body. Physical stress can result in physical problems, but also in chemical or mental/emotional problems.

Chemical Stress

Chemicals from any source can affect body chemistry and cause stress. This includes dietary and nutritional imbalances such as too much or too little food or nutrients, excess caffeine or drugs, and ingestion of chemicals from food and water supplies. Other sources of chemical stress include those in the air — second-hand smoke, indoor and outdoor air pollution and many others. Chemical stresses can cause indigestion, fatigue, insomnia, or even physical and emotional problems.

Mental and Emotional Stress

Mental and emotional stress is the type with which most people are familiar. This includes tension, anxiety and depression. Mental stress may contribute to pain, moods of anxiety or depression, and loss of enthusiasm or motivation, and can lead to physical and chemical problems as well. Mental stress also affects cognition, including sensation, perception, learning, concept formation and decision-making.

Stress can come from anywhere: your job, family, other people, your emotions, infections, allergic reactions, physical trauma and exertion, even the weather. Remember, not all stress is negative. Since it evokes a reaction in the body, the outcome may be a positive one — the benefit of exercise is one example. By mildly stressing your body, over time and through adaptation, your body performs better. But that same stressor — your workout — can become negative if you go too far beyond the body's ability to recover from it.

Usually people are stressed in more than one area, and frequently by all three types. And, stress is cumulative. The response to a physical stress from the weekend's yard work may be amplified by Monday's chemical stress of too much coffee or the wrong foods, further compounded with a family-related mental stress on Tuesday and another with the boss on Wednesday. All of this will affect your performance at an important meeting on Friday.

The weather is also a potential stressor, with certain people more vulnerable. Weather stress may affect us physically, chemically or mentally. Extremes in temperature or humidity, very low barometric pressure, and the sun are stressors. Seasonal Affective Disorder (SAD) is a good example of how the weather at certain times of year (typically in the fall and winter) can have a dramatic effect on many people.

Some people accumulate so much stress they lose track of it, which becomes more of a stress. The first thing to do with stress is to make sure you're aware of it. The remedy? Write it all down.

Making Your Stress List

Being more aware of your physical, chemical and mental stress is a big step for improving health. Reducing or eliminating individual stresses is easier if you write them down on paper. On a page, make three columns, one each for physical, chemical and mental stresses. In each category, write down your stresses. This may take several days to complete since you probably won't think of all your different stresses right away. When you're done, prioritize by placing the biggest stress of each category on top. Then, work on reducing or eliminating one stress at a time. Or, if you can handle it, work on one stress at a time from each category. Reducing or eliminating unnecessary stress from your life will give your body a better chance to cope with other stresses you may not be able to change right now.

As you make your list put a star by the stresses over which you have some control. This may include unhealthy eating habits like rushing or skipping your meals, drinking too much coffee or not taking time to exercise.

Simply draw a line through those stresses that you can't control. If there's nothing you can do about them anyway, don't worry about them for now. Many people expend lots of energy on stresses they can't or won't do anything about. This may include job stress or the weather, though in reality, almost any stress can be modified or eliminated — it's just a question of how far you're willing to go for optimal health. As time goes on, you may want to reconsider some of the items you've crossed off. You'll realize that changing jobs is a must, or moving to a more compatible climate is necessary for your health.

Once you can "see" your stress listed on paper, it will be easier to manage. Start with your starred stresses first, because you have control over them — not that it's always easy. Circle the three biggest stresses from the starred list and begin to work on them. You may be able to improve on some and totally eliminate others. Some will require habit changes. It's a big task, but one that will return great benefits. When you've succeeded in eliminating or modifying each one, cross it off your list and circle the three next most stressful ones, so you always have three to work on.

In addition to your stress list, you're probably familiar with other strategies for dealing with stress, though you may not use them. Here's a reminder:

- Learn to say "no" when asked to do something you really don't want to do. Ask yourself if you really want to do this.

- Decide not to waste your time worrying about the past or the future. That's not to say you should ignore the past or not plan for the future. Live in the present.

- Learn some relaxation techniques, and perform them regularly. The most powerful one is respiratory biofeedback described previously. An easy walk by yourself can also be a great way to relax.

- When you're concerned about something, talk it over with someone you trust.

- Simplify your life. Start by eliminating trivia. Ask yourself: "Is this really important?"

- Prioritize your busy schedule; do the most important things first. But don't neglect the enjoyable things. Before getting out of bed in the morning, ask yourself: "What fun things do I have planned for today?"

- Know your passion and pursue it.

What's most important about stress is that too much of it interferes with rest. Or more accurately, recovering from excess stress requires more rest. If you don't get enough rest, usually in the form of sleep, the effects of stress will continue accumulating. One of the questions to ask yourself is whether you're getting enough sleep, considering the amount of stress you have. As you will see, one of the symptoms of excess stress is insomnia.

By learning to take control of the various types of stress in your life, you can improve the quality of your life, reduce the risk of dysfunction and disease, and also help your adrenal glands regulate stress. Maintaining proper adrenal function is central to optimal fitness and health.

Case History
Dave had numerous complaints — physical, chemical and mental. A Wall Street executive, he was building a new home and had spring and fall allergies that nearly incapacitated him each year. Dave spent more than two weeks making and pondering his stress list. After discussing all the issues with family and friends, he decided to make some changes. Dave and his family sold their partially built house, moved to a nicer climate, and he secured a job with less stress. Though the pay was less, so were the taxes and other stresses. Within six months, Dave felt 15 years younger. Even his family was healthier, and they felt closer.

The Adrenal Glands
No matter what type of stress you encounter during your life journey — be it physical, chemical or mental/emotional — your body has an efficient mechanism for coping. This is the important job of the adrenal glands. On the top of each kidney, these small glands work with

The General Adaptation Syndrome

Our knowledge about stress and adrenal function began in the early 1900s, when famous stress-research pioneer Hans Selye began to piece together the common triad of signs resulting from excess adrenal stress. They include adrenal-gland enlargement, depressed immunity and intestinal dysfunction. Selye eventually showed how the adrenals react when confronted with excess stress. This General Adaptation Syndrome has three distinct stages.

Stage 1: The first stage begins with the alarm reaction, in which there is an increase in adrenal hormone production. This is an attempt by the adrenals to battle the increased stress. If it is successful, adrenal function returns to normal. During this stage, a variety of mild symptoms may occur: spotty tiredness during the day, mild allergies or even some nagging back, knee or foot pain. If, over time, the adrenals fail to meet the needs of the body to combat the stress, they enter the second stage, called the resistance stage.

Stage 2: During this period, the adrenal glands themselves get larger through a process called hypertrophy. Since the increased hormone production of the first stage couldn't counter the stress, the glands enlarge in an attempt make even more cortisol to do the same. During this stage, more advanced symptoms may occur, including fatigue, insomnia and more serious back, knee or foot pain. Most people with stress problems are stuck in this stage. But if the stress persists and is still not controlled, the adrenals eventually can enter the third stage, called exhaustion.

Stage 3: If a person enters this stage he or she is exhausted. The adrenal glands are unable to adapt to stress and produce adequate levels of hormones, including cortisol. The person is usually seriously ill, physically, chemically or mentally.

the nervous system to regulate the important coping mechanisms, including the "fight or flight" reactions. The adrenal glands accomplish their work through the production of certain hormones, making them not only essential for stress coping and optimal human performance, but also for life itself. These hormones help with stress regulation, sex and reproduction, growth, aging, cellular repair, electrolyte balance and blood-sugar control.

The nervous system also helps in coping with stress. This occurs through messages sent throughout the brain and nervous system, and through two other important stress hormones, epinephrine and norepinephrine.

Cortisol is the key adrenal stress hormone, and commonly measured by simple blood and saliva tests. When your body is under high stress, cortisol levels can increase dramatically, and when the stress passes it returns to normal levels. In chronic stress states — the continuation of stress without relief — high cortisol levels can become dangerous. This can adversely affect the brain, especially memory, create blood sugar problems, reduce fat-burning, suppress immune function, lowering the body's defense against not just cold and flu but any infections, and cause intestinal distress. Long-standing stress can result in a "burning out" of adrenal function, with a serious loss of normal hormone production. In this state, cortisol levels become dangerously low, along with other hormones made by the adrenals.

The sex hormones, including estrogens, progesterone and testosterone, are also important adrenal hormones that help both males and females maintain proper sexual function and reproductive health. The adrenals also make dehydroepiandrosterone, or DHEA, which is the precursor to the estrogens, and testosterone.

This discussion is not about adrenal disease, rather, the gray area between normal adrenal function and disease. Addison's disease occurs when the adrenal glands are unable to produce sufficient cortisol to sustain life. It can occur in men and women of all age groups; symptoms include severe weight loss, muscle weakness, fatigue, low blood pressure, and sometimes darkening of the skin. The disease is also called adrenal insufficiency, or hypocortisolism.

Are You 'Stressed Out?'

Excess adrenal stress — or an insufficient adrenal response to adapt to stress — is a common problem. It is often the result of chronically overstimulated adrenal glands, in some cases to the point of exhaustion. The popular lingo is usually the notion that you're "stressed-out." If you're in business, "burn-out" is the common name, with "nervous breakdown" used in the past. If you're an athlete, it's called "overtraining." Whatever the name, it's essentially the same problem of adrenal dysfunction, with serious implications for fitness and health that can dramatically reduce quality of life.

Ten common symptoms of adrenal dysfunction are listed below. Check off any that pertain to you. They can be caused by other imbalances in the body. But taken together, they make up the most common symptoms of adrenal dysfunction.

- ❏ **Low energy.** This is common especially in the afternoon, but could happen anytime, or all the time. The fatigue can be physical, mental or both. When the adrenals are too stressed, the body uses more sugar for energy, but can't access fat very well for energy use. This can significantly limit your energy.

- ❏ **Dizziness upon standing.** Standing up from a seated or lying position can make you dizzy because not enough blood is getting to the head quickly enough. Check your blood pressure while lying down, and then immediately after you stand. If you suffer from adrenal dysfunction, you will notice the systolic blood pressure (the first number) doesn't rise normally — it should be higher when you're standing by about 6 to 8 mm.

- ❏ **Eyes sensitive to bright light.** Adrenal stress often causes light sensitivity in your eyes. You may need to wear sunglasses or have difficulty with night driving because of the oncoming headlights. You may even misinterpret this as having bad night vision. Some people find their nearsightedness (ability to see distances) improves after improving adrenal function.

❏ **Asthma and allergies.** Whether you call it exercise-induced asthma, food allergies or seasonal allergies, they are similar symptoms of adrenal dysfunction.

❏ **Mechanical imbalance.** Problems in the low back, knee, foot and ankle are often associated with adrenal problems. These areas can become mechanically unstable and produce symptoms such as low-back pain, sciatica and excess pronation in the foot, leading to foot and ankle problems.

❏ **Stress-related syndromes.** The problems referred to as burnout, stressed-out, overtraining (overexercising) and nervous breakdown are almost always the result of adrenal exhaustion. While occasionally these problems become serious enough to warrant medication or hospitalization, adrenal dysfunction occurs long before this point.

❏ **Blood-sugar-handling stress.** With adrenal dysfunction, the body is unable to properly control blood sugar. Symptoms include constantly feeling hungry, being irritable before meals or if meals are delayed, and having strong cravings for sweets or caffeine.

❏ **Insomnia.** Many people with adrenal dysfunction fall asleep easily (often because of exhaustion) but wake in the middle of the night with difficulty getting back to sleep. This may be due to high levels of cortisol occurring at the wrong time (levels should be low during sleeping hours). Many people say they wake up in the night to urinate. But it's usually the adrenal problem that awakens them, and then they get the urge to urinate.

❏ **Diminished sexual drive.** This is a common symptom of adrenal dysfunction due to low levels of the hormone DHEA, which makes estrogen and testosterone. (Low levels of these hormones can also adversely affect the strength of bones and muscles.)

❏ **Seasonal Affective Disorder (SAD).** This is a common problem, especially in the fall and winter. As the hours of daylight lessen and the temperature drops, many people go into a mild state of hibernation. The metabolism slows, and the body and mind become sluggish, sometimes resulting in a mild or moderate depression. (This corresponds with a combination of stresses: the weather, lack of sunlight and even the start of the holiday season — people don't eat well, are less active, and weight gain is common.)

Recognizing these 10 common symptoms of adrenal dysfunction can be useful in your self-assessment. You may also want to test some of your adrenal-hormone levels with the help of a professional. The best test for adrenal hormones measures cortisol and DHEA, and is usually performed over the course of a typical day and evening using four saliva test samples, rather than just a single test.

With an awareness of the signs and symptoms of adrenal stress, you can make some appropriate lifestyle changes to improve adrenal function and possibly solve many of your problems. Earlier I discussed the importance of making your stress list. Now, let's look at some of the other factors related to improving adrenal function: diet, exercise and lifestyle. Many of these have been addressed in earlier chapters but presented here in the context of adrenal dysfunction.

Diet and Adrenal Stress

One of the most important dietary factors related to adrenal stress is the consumption of refined carbohydrate and sugar. This includes hidden sugars in many foods. How much is too much? Perform the Two-Week Test if you're not sure.

Caffeine is a common source of adrenal stimulation, a main reason people consume it. Coffee, tea and colas are the main sources. If you have an adrenal problem, assess your caffeine intake. For many, no caffeine is best; for others, a single cup or two of coffee or tea may be tolerable. You must determine, as objectively as possible by listening to your body, how much caffeine you can tolerate.

Always eat a healthy breakfast. This includes protein but void of refined carbohydrates. An egg-based meal can be the cornerstone of an ideal breakfast.

People with adrenal stress often need to snack between the three main meals, even every two hours in the early stages of recovery. Healthy snacking habits were discussed in Chapter 20. Low-carbohydrate snacks include almonds and cashews, cheese, vegetables and hard-boiled eggs. Avoid fruit juice.

Nutrients for Adrenal Stress

Your nutritional needs may vary with adrenal stress. These include factors to help the immune system, gut and the adrenal glands themselves. Since the hormonal system is very complex, it's recommended that you seek the input of a health-care professional to correct a hormonal imbalance. Below are some possible supplemental nutrient needs:

- For many types of adrenal stress, especially those that cause insomnia, zinc may be useful. Studies show this important mineral can help lower high cortisol levels that accompany adrenal stress. Taken right before bed, for example, zinc may improve sleep patterns. A metallic taste in your mouth may mean that you're taking too much zinc, so be careful with zinc supplementation.

- Choline is a nutrient commonly needed by some people with adrenal stress, in part due to the relationship of choline with the nervous system. Individuals who are always on the go, overworked and trying to do too much are examples of those who may benefit from choline. Small amounts several times a day may be very helpful. The best source of choline in the diet is egg yolks. Those with asthma symptoms generally need even more choline.

- Intestinal dysfunction almost always accompanies adrenal stress. This issue is discussed in Chapter 29.

Exercise and Adrenal Stress

In general, easy aerobic activity is helpful for all except the person in the end stage of adrenal exhaustion. In this case rest may be most important until adrenal function begins to improve. Anaerobic exercise can worsen adrenal problems at any stage.

If you do not already exercise, a 20- to 30-minute easy walk, five times per week, is a great adrenal therapy. If you already work out, maintain easy aerobic exercise, such as walking. It will build the small aerobic muscle fibers, promoting more fat-burning and increasing circulation, both of which will help adrenal function.

Avoid all anaerobic workouts, including weight-lifting and any exercise that raises the heart rate above your aerobic level. Once adrenal function is improved, anaerobic exercise can be resumed, though the balance of aerobic and anaerobic exercise must be maintained as discussed in previous chapters. In addition to these factors, other lifestyle issues are worth considering:

- A relaxing massage, such as a Swedish massage, can help reduce high cortisol levels. Avoid massages that cause pain, which could increase stress.

- Sunlight on the skin and through the eyes is important for proper adrenal function and can help improve dysfunction. Do not stare directly into the sun; just spending time outdoors provides sufficient photo stimulation through the skin and eyes. Natural, full-spectrum light from the sun can help the brain, which influences adrenal function. Window glass, prescription and non-prescription glasses and contact lenses can filter out the stimulating part of the light spectrum. If you normally are exposed to little or no sun, take a walk during your lunch break to get some natural light (even on a cloudy day). For indoor use, consider replacing your regular light bulbs and tubes in locations where you spend considerable time with full spectrum lights.

- Evaluate your sleeping habits. Are you getting at least seven to eight hours each night? If not, you may need more. Adrenal stress increases the need for recovery. Decide what changes are needed to ensure that you are getting enough sleep.

- Research shows that enjoyable music can lower high cortisol levels. Play music while in your car, at work or at home. Choose music you like but avoid the radio with its stressful commercials and commentary. Play the music you liked during the more stress-free and happiest times of your life.

- Various meditation methods can counter stress, especially respiratory biofeedback discussed in Chapter 28.

Other Natural Hormones

Hormones play a major role in your physical, chemical and mental well-being. The key to optimal hormonal performance is balance, and adrenal health is primary. Three key hormones, important for and produced by both men and women, include the estrogens, testosterone and progesterone. As you age, and with increased stress, the production of these hormones is diminished. This occurs especially when cortisol rises, diminishing the production of DHEA, and subsequently, diminishing estrogen, testosterone and progesterone.

If you think your hormones are diminishing, the first step is to assess them. Salivary hormone tests are performed by many healthcare professionals. If your hormones are not balanced (some may be high while others are low), the next step is to consider all the adrenal-related issues discussed in this chapter. Replacing your natural hormones with synthetic versions has been a topic of major controversy due to dangerous side effects, and should not be a first option. Many people can restore normal hormone balance by improving adrenal gland function, which usually includes other issues discussed in this book. When this is not sufficient, natural hormone supplements may be necessary.

Estrogen

This most well known of hormones is actually a group of about 20 compounds. The most important estrogens are estrone, estradiol and estriol. The different estrogens have unique roles in the body. For example, estradiol is the most stimulating to the breast, and is the estrogen related to increased risk of breast cancer. Estriol protects against breast cancer. Normal production of both by the body is the right balance. A variety of benefits are attributed to the effects of natural estrogens, including prevention of hot flashes, better memory and concentration, slowing of the aging process, and reduced depression and anxiety.

Synthetic estradiol (Premarin) is the estrogen that places you at high risk for breast cancer. This is due to the fact that it's not broken down in the liver as quickly as your own natural estrogens (affecting the cells for a longer time). Premarin, made from the urine of pregnant horses, simply doesn't function exactly like the estrogens made in the human body. In addition to natural estradiol, other natural estrogens have synthetic companions and are marketed under various brand names.

One of the common risks of taking synthetic estrogen is the higher dosage compared to what your body would normally produce. The most common symptom of too much estrogen in your system is water retention. This can lead to breast tenderness and swelling, weight gain and headaches. Excess estrogen can also lower blood sugar and increase your cravings for sweets. Too much estrogen also increases your risk of uterine cancer and gall bladder disease.

While the idea of synthetic estrogen replacement is often "sold" to patients by touting the benefits of building strong bones, estrogen doesn't actually do this. Rather, it decreases the rate of bone loss that occurs naturally throughout life. The hormones that have the greatest impact on new bone growth — something your body is always doing — are progesterone and testosterone.

Progesterone and Testosterone

Unlike estrogen, which is a group of hormones, progesterone is the only hormone in its class. Progesterone has many functions in the body. It improves sleep, builds bone mass, protects against breast and uterine cancer, improves carbohydrate tolerance, helps burn fat, prevents water retention, increases sex drive and in many people has a calming effect on the nervous system.

Provera is a synthetic version of progesterone, one that is given to many women. However, it doesn't have the same functions as the natural hormone. While natural progesterone acts like a diuretic, Provera can increase salt and water retention, and increase body fat. Too much of this synthetic hormone can cause bloating, depression, fatigue, increased hair on the body, and increased weight gain. Provera can also cause your body to diminish its own production of natural progesterone, forcing you to rely more on outside sources. Other synthetics can cause birth defects, epilepsy, asthma and heart problems.

It's important to note that both estrogen and progesterone work together. In a real sense, they balance each other when in their natural state. Taking one form without the balance of the other often creates stress.

Testosterone is also a naturally occurring hormone made by both men and women. This hormone is important for healing, helps build and maintain muscles and bones, increases sex drive and overall energy, and is a very important hormone for other areas of the metabolism. The synthetic version is methyltestosterone, with side effects including hormonal imbalance, intestinal distress, increased cholesterol, hair loss, depression, anxiety and others.

Getting Yours Naturally

The ideal scenario is to have your body make the types and amounts of hormones necessary for you. That amount varies from day to day and year to year (even from minute to minute). If reduced health interferes with this delicate mechanism, imbalances can occur. I can't emphasize enough that preventing and correcting hormone imbalance by improving adrenal function and overall fitness and health is the most effective and best first option.

If you have signs and symptoms related to hormone imbalance, measuring your hormone levels, by testing the blood and/or saliva, is very important. A re-evaluation of any abnormal test results will help you know whether improved lifestyle habits or any replacement therapy is successful.

If you're still producing too little hormone after trying all the healthy habits discussed in previous chapters (especially balancing dietary carbohydrate, fat and protein), taking natural hormones to

Plants to the Rescue

Another potential natural hormone therapy is to use natural plants. These are sometimes effective in people with relatively minor hormone imbalance. Many plants contain natural hormones, and a variety of products are made from them in concentrated forms. These include wild yams, soy products and licorice root. However, there are two possible problems with these products, which have become very popular. Their levels of hormones are generally very low; and some unscrupulous companies make products with hardly any or no measurable hormones. In the case of soy, there could be unwanted side effects. And in the case of licorice, it could raise your cortisol levels — a problem that may already exist and be the cause of hormone imbalance.

replace what you're not making may be the next best option. It's important to ask your health-care professional about these alternatives as many are by prescription. For more information, contact the Women's International Pharmacy (800-279-5708, www.womensinternational.com), Hopewell Pharmacy (800-792-6670, www.hopewell-rx.com) or other reliable sources.

Some non-prescription products are also available. Pro-Gest, for example, is a natural progesterone cream that can be absorbed through the skin rather than taken by mouth (your liver breaks down much of the natural hormone taken orally). For those who require both natural estrogen and progesterone, a product called OstaDerm cream is also a non-prescription preparation of both natural hormones.

For menopause, premenstrual syndrome, or other hormone-related imbalances, the use of natural hormones can improve your quality of life. What's most important is to understand that no one has to live with the pain, displeasure and discomfort that too many doctors have told patients are normal with aging.

Case History

Sally was in her early 40s and had a variety of hormone-related symptoms, including hot flashes, insomnia and body-fat increase, all beginning over the previous two years. Her doctor wanted her to start taking synthetic hormones, but she was uneasy since her family history included breast cancer. My first choice was to try to get Sally's adrenal function improved, as tests showed her cortisol and DHEA levels to be far from normal. After several months of making lifestyle changes, Sally's symptoms improved by about 50 percent. At this time, I recommended she begin using a natural progesterone cream, once per day after showering. Within three months, Sally began feeling better, and within six months, felt more like she did when she was 30.

Stress-induced adrenal dysfunction is one of the major problems associated with a wide range of fitness and health problems. Improving adrenal function can quickly resolve many common signs and symptoms that reduce quality of life.

32

The Overfat Epidemic

Weight loss is a primary concern of most people. Trillions of dollars have been spend on it without real success. Millions of dollars are spent each year to research the problem of being overweight. The result is a threatening of the industrialized world with an epidemic of overfat people. We can discuss how much body fat is too much, the definitions of obesity and other commonly discussed issues, but the fact is, too much body fat is unhealthy. Rather than dancing around the issues of percent body fat and the latest definitions of obesity, let's just call the problem what it is: overfat.

By 2015, scientists say, 75 percent of Americans will be overfat, with the rest of the world not far behind. In the U.S., women 20-34 years old are the fastest growing group of overfat people. And in some populations — individuals with darker skin — the numbers of overfat people are generally much worse. For example, more than 80 percent of black women are overfat. At one time the overfat problem affected adults almost exclusively. But today, overfat children are everywhere.

The primary problem is simple; for most people it's the overconsumption of sugar and refined carbohydrates. It's not necessarily the overconsumption of calories of these foods, but even so-called low-calorie sugar foods can overproduce insulin with the result of storing more of this low-fat food as body fat. Companies creating these foods, and those selling them, are the next targets of government and lawyers — much like the attack on cigarette companies of recent decades.

Most of the issues about being overweight fail to address the problem. It's not about weight, it's about being overfat. Excess body fat is unhealthy for two reasons. First, it's unhealthy because of the reason it accumulated in the first place — for most, it's unhealthy eating habits, for example, as I just noted regarding sugar and refined carbohydrates. Second, stored body fat produces inflammatory chemicals that are a very serious threat to overall health. Chronic inflammation is the first step in the process of development of most chronic diseases, from Alzheimer's and cancer to diabetes and heart disease.

What is Weight?

Most people consider excess body weight and body fat as synonymous. But this is untrue: what most really want to do is lose body fat. We live in a weight-conscious society, and stepping on the scale each morning is a powerful ritual, one difficult to break. Most of the weight the scale measures is water, and most of this water is in the muscles and other body areas, not fat. Body fat weighs much less. However, body fat takes up much more space than water. Everyone knows this: as we gain or lose fat, our clothes fit differently. In fact, many of the patients I helped lose body fat often didn't lose weight — and some actually gained weight while getting healthy and losing inches off their waist. As body fat is reduced, improved muscle function adds more weight, a healthy sign. So if we want to address the real issue — reducing body fat — the best way to evaluate is by measuring body size.

There are many ways to measure body size, and even percent body fat. Many weight-loss programs sell various gadgets for determining this issue. But in keeping with simplifying the stress in your life, my suggestion is to avoid the task of trying to focus on these more detailed measurements — and avoid the risk of creating a new obsession of measuring yourself. The most simple and practical way to calculate changes in body fat is by periodically measuring your waist with a tape measure. Do this at the level of the umbilicus, the belly button. No other approach will provide you with more information about what you need to do — either reduce or maintain body fat levels.

For most people, it's body fat that should be the focus. Reducing body fat should be done in a healthy way, and fortunately, for the majority of people, this is not difficult to accomplish. Essentially, this whole book is about burning body fat, so this chapter will refer the reader to other chapters for more detailed discussions of certain aspects of fat-burning. For most people, this begins with the Two-Week Test described earlier. In that chapter I suggest weighing yourself before and after the test only, just for reference.

Calorie Restriction

Restricting calories as a means of losing body weight is the most common approach used in the weight-loss industry. And 95 percent of those who go on a calorie-restricted diet will fail. This includes many who lose weight initially. Most will gain it back — plus more — in the end. Moreover, many will not lose significant body fat but instead will lose muscle.

By performing a computerized dietary analysis on almost every patient I've seen in practice, it's clear that most people who restrict calories also restricted nutrients. This results in a loss of health and human performance. Dehydration, nutrient loss, muscle and bone loss, lowered metabolism that shifts to more sugar- and less fat-burning and other health issues are most often the real result of weight loss from calorie restriction. In some, the result has been an eating disorder that can be even more difficult to treat.

Throughout this book I've emphasized the importance of fat-burning — especially how reducing sugar and refined carbohydrates increases it, and how building the aerobic system increases it. By increasing fat-burning, you'll lose inches on your waist, reduce body fat, have unlimited energy, and not just look and feel fit and healthy but actually live it.

The ABCs of Burning Body Fat

This is the shortest chapter in the book because most of what I've written is a review of the other chapters. For almost everyone who has too much body fat, following these three steps will result in the loss of significant body fat (there will always be a very few exceptions with unusual metabolic disorders or other rare problems).

    A: **Perform the Two-Week Test.** Read about carbohydrates and sugars, perform the test and determine your tolerance to carbohydrate foods.

B: **Balance your fats.** Don't avoid them, unless they're bad. Eat sufficient amounts of good fats.

C: **Build your aerobic system through easy exercise.** For most people, walking is sufficient.

By focusing on improving health and aerobic fitness, there is almost always an appropriate loss of body fat.

Thyroid Troubles

Thyroid dysfunction may be a problem in some people who have difficulty losing body fat. Low thyroid function leads to symptoms that include mental and physical fatigue, increased body fat, depression and skin problems (especially cracking around the heels and on the hands). Hair loss is also common, especially thinning of the lateral one-third of the eyebrow. The first step is to evaluate thyroid function through blood tests; free T3 and T4, and TSH levels. If these are not normal, thyroid antibodies should be measured. But blood tests don't always show the relatively minor functional thyroid problems. Saliva tests may be more important for detecting subclinical thyroid dysfunction. You can also take your temperature — those with low thyroid function usually have low temperatures. Below-normal temperatures — less than about 98.6° Fahrenheit or 37° Celcius — may indicate thyroid dysfunction. (Note that NSAIDS — nonsteroidal anti-inflammatory drugs — including aspirin, ibuprofen and others, can also disturb metabolism and decrease body temperature.)

As you improve the quality of your diet and build the aerobic system, and fat-burning begins to increase, thyroid function will improve too. This will be reflected in more normal body temperature and improvements in any other abnormal blood or saliva tests.

33

Chronic Inflammation: The Other Epidemic

Inflammation is typically thought of as swelling, pain or discomfort, perhaps in your joints, sinuses or intestines. But for many people chronic inflammation occurs without symptoms and may be the cause of other health problems. A full spectrum of disorders is associated with chronic inflammation — from severe functional problems such as fatigue, hormonal imbalance and reduced immunity, to serious diseases such as osteoporosis, heart disease and cancer. Balancing fat intake is one of the key factors to controlling chronic inflammation.

There are two forms of inflammation — acute and chronic. Acute inflammation is a normal healthy action, helping to heal more than just that little cut on our finger. Without it, you would not recover from a day at the office, your easy walk, or even the minor bumps and bruises you acquire during your life. But acute inflammation can also be triggered more significantly by various traumas such as a fall, more intense exercise such as weight-lifting, infections, toxins in food and air, synthetic hormones and excess stress.

There are three important functions of acute inflammation. One is the first step in the healing or repair process after some physical or chemical injury or stress, no matter how minor. The second is that it prevents the spread of damaged cells that could cause secondary problems in other areas of the body. A local infection, for example, can be contained due to the inflammatory response, instead of causing a bodywide infection. Third, inflammation rids the body of damaged and dead cells.

Normally, the inflammatory cycle is almost like an "on-off" switch. It's turned on by inflammatory chemicals when it is needed for healing and repair. Then it's turned off by anti-inflammatory chemicals when it's not needed. It's when these anti-inflammatory chemicals are not present in sufficient quantity, or there's too much inflammatory-causing stress, that the switch stays on. The outcome is chronic inflammation.

Chronic Inflammation

When inflammation continues into the chronic state, many health problems can begin developing. This may include those all-too-familiar "itis" conditions such as tendinitis, colitis, sinusitis and arthritis. Chronic inflammation is also a precursor to ulceration, and it could ultimately lead to disease.

For some people, the presence of inflammation is obvious. But most people with chronic inflammation are not aware of it because the signs and symptoms may not be apparent. Therefore, some type of evaluation is important. The following survey may help guide you in determining your potential for inflammation. Check the items that pertain to you:

- ❏ Do you eat restaurant, take-out or prepared food daily?

- ❏ Do you consume milk, cream, butter or cheese regularly?

- ❏ Do you consume corn, soy, safflower or peanut oils regularly?

- ❏ Do you consume margarine or products that contain hydrogenated or partially hydrogenated oils regularly?

- ❏ Is your diet low in fresh salmon, sardines and other cold-water fish?

- ❏ Do you have a history of atherosclerosis, stroke or heart disease?

- ❏ Do you have a history of osteoporosis?

- ❏ Do you have a history of ulcer or cancer?

- ❏ Do you have a history of "itis" conditions such as arthritis, colitis, tendinitis, etc.?

- ❏ Do you have allergies, asthma or recurring infections?

- ❏ Do you have chronic fatigue?

❏ Do you have increased body fat?

❏ Do you perform weekly anaerobic exercise, such as weight-lifting, hard training or competition?

❏ Do you perform regular repetitive activity (jogging, cycling, walking, typing, etc.)?

Even if you check only one or two of the above items, it indicates an increased chance of having chronic inflammation.

A simple blood test can confirm the presence of inflammation. The C-reactive protein (CRP) test is the most accurate screen for inflammation and can detect very low levels. This test can also predict future risk of coronary heart disease and stroke even in otherwise healthy individuals. The best suggestion is to have a CRP performed regularly, when other blood tests are ordered. If the result is not normal, retest every six months until it's normal. CRP levels should be lower than 1.0 mg/L, which is the lowest risk of developing cardiovascular disease. Between 1.0 and 3.0 mg/L, a person has average risk and CRP levels higher than 3.0 mg/L are associated with a high risk.

Other blood tests include the erythrocyte sedimentation rate (ESR). This common blood test for inflammation can be performed when blood is taken for other tests, or with a finger prick. A complete blood count measures white blood cells and may also indicate inflammation. Compare your results to the reference ranges given by the lab.

Diet and Inflammation

Many of the chemicals involved in both inflammation and anti-inflammation are heavily influenced by your diet. This was discussed in Chapter 10 and is reviewed here because of its importance. The four items below can have a dramatic effect on reducing unwanted inflammation.

• Balance your intake of dietary fats as discussed in Chapter 10. To accomplish this it may be necessary to supplement your diet with EPA from fish oil.

• Make sure you have all the nutrients necessary for maintaining balanced fats, including vitamins B6, E, C and niacin and the minerals magnesium and zinc. These are best obtained from a healthy diet.

- Avoid specific foods and lifestyle factors that disturb the balance of fats. These include trans fat, refined carbohydrates and sugars, and overexercise.

- Certain foods can fight inflammation. Ginger and turmeric are powerful foods that can help control inflammation. These are common spices used in many types of foods. While fresh turmeric is more difficult to find in stores, fresh ginger is common. Ginger can be used in salads, or to make tea, or is added to many dishes for its pungent flavor. And it can be pickled. Developing a habit of using ginger regularly in your meals can be very helpful in controlling inflammation. Turmeric is in the ginger family, and probably on your spice shelf. It's commonly used as a natural coloring agent, and is a major ingredient in curry powder.

Many people eat citrus fruit but toss the peel. They are throwing out some of the most important nutritional factors. The oil in citrus peel contains limonene, a powerful phytonutrient. When eating the fruit, eat the skin, or at least the white parts. This is more enjoyable when the fruit is tree-ripened, which makes for a much sweeter skin.

Foods in the onion family can also help reduce inflammation, especially garlic and onions. In our culture, garlic and onions are often avoided due to the odor after eating them. But both have great therapeutic benefits and should be part of your daily diet, even if it's just in your evening meal. Other foods in the onion family include shallots and chives.

Functional Illness

Chronic inflammation that's allowed to continue unchecked can lead to a full spectrum of functional problems, such as fatigue, hormonal imbalance and reduced immunity. Fatigue may be among the more common results of chronic inflammation. Other problems associated with chronic inflammation include:

- **Lowered immunity.** Indicated by frequent infections, including colds and flu, and yeast and fungal infections such as Candida. Asthma, allergies and other issues also may be due to low immunity and chronic inflammation.

- **Hormonal imbalance.** This can include many aspects of the hormonal system, especially the adrenal stress hormones, reducing your ability to cope with stress. Sex hormones — estrogen, progesterone and testosterone — can also be adversely affected, resulting in diminished sex drive, reproductive function and muscle and bone health. Reduced thyroid function can also result due to inhibition of thyroid-stimulating hormone.

- **Nervous-system imbalance.** This includes increased activity of the sympathetic nervous system, potentially leading to increased tension, rising blood pressure, disturbed blood sugar, anxiety or depression, or other problems.

- **Digestive distress.** Among the problems that can result are poor digestion, gas formation, heartburn and various inflammatory conditions such as colitis and ileitis. Poor absorption of nutrients can be another result, creating an entire series of potential problems throughout the body.

- **Chronic pain.** Inflammation produces pain-stimulating chemicals throughout the body. This also results in a reduced pain threshold.

- **Cataracts.** Another common condition that develops with age is cataracts, and inflammation plays a major role in the development of this eye disease. Chronic inflammation has been shown to predispose healthy individuals to future risk of age-related cataracts.

- **Gingivitis and periodontal disease.** These oral conditions are also associated with inflammation, and may be a silent cause of chronic bodywide inflammation.

- **Hair loss.** Loss of hair may be associated with inflammation in the scalp, specifically the hair follicles.

Chronic Diseases

In the long term, chronic inflammation can lead to more serious diseases. It is now considered a major risk factor for cardiovascular disease, for example. A variety of other disease states may be an end result of chronic inflammation, including ulcers and cancer, atherosclerosis, stroke, osteoporosis and even type 2 diabetes.

Other common diseases associated with inflammation have "itis" at the ends of their names: arthritis (inflammation of the joints), colitis (inflammation of the colon), tendinitis (inflammation of a tendon), etc. Even chronic fatigue syndrome and anorexia may be part of the chronic inflammation problem.

Balancing fats is the key to maintaining the balance of inflammatory chemicals. This may mean making some changes in your diet, nutrition and lifestyle, or finding ways to reduce stress levels. Controlling your inflammation is an important step forward for your health. Not only will it improve your quality of life now, it will also pay off bigger benefits later in life by warding off dangerous, life-threatening illnesses.

34

The Big Picture of Heart Disease

Heart disease is a leading cause of death in the United States, and a major problem throughout the industrialized world. Despite the abundance of low-fat and low-cholesterol foods and diets, the numbers of new cases, and deaths, keep growing.

Chronic inflammation may be the most common cause of heart disease. If you have chronic inflammation, your risk for having a heart attack is doubled. Studies show that the more inflammation — as indicated with a simple blood test (C-reactive protein as discussed in the previous chapter) — the greater your risk of having a heart attack. In fact, each of the many stages of cardiovascular disease is associated with inflammatory factors. In addition, there is a strong association between chronic inflammation and other cardiovascular problems including sudden cardiac death, peripheral arterial disease, stroke and other conditions.

Of course, other unhealthy lifestyle factors significantly increase the risk of heart disease. These include smoking, being overfat, hypertension and others. Diabetes, an end-stage problem of carbohydrate intolerance, is a major risk factor. These problems, however, contribute to heart disease because they also are associated with and/or increase chronic inflammation. Aerobic exercise is also very important for the heart; inactivity puts you at nearly as great a risk as smoking.

Cholesterol

One of the most misunderstood subjects related to heart disease is cholesterol. Abnormally high levels of cholesterol can also be a risk factor for heart disease, although your total cholesterol is not the best — or only — measure for heart-disease risk. Many people who die of heart disease have normal total cholesterol numbers, and many with high cholesterol never develop heart disease.

Perhaps the greatest misconception about cholesterol is that eating foods containing it significantly raises levels in the blood. In truth, most studies have shown that eating cholesterol does not alone substantially increase blood-cholesterol levels. Moreover, some studies show that not eating cholesterol can prompt your body to make more — and that eating eggs can improve your cholesterol numbers!

While there is a correlation between higher total cholesterol in the blood and incidences of heart attacks, evaluating cardiac risk calls for a complete fasting blood-lipid profile that measures at least total, HDL and LDL cholesterol, and triglycerides.

The most important thing to know about cholesterol is that cholesterol itself isn't "bad," but rather something to be kept in balance. It's also important to understand that most of the cholesterol in the bloodstream is actually made by the liver. If you eat more cholesterol, your body prompts the liver to make less of it. But if you take in less, your liver makes more. That's why many people on a low-cholesterol diet still have high blood-cholesterol levels.

Actually, all cells in the body — including those of the heart — make cholesterol every day. That's because cholesterol is necessary for many essential processes that keep us healthy. For example, the outer surfaces of cells contain cholesterol, which helps regulate which chemicals enter and exit. Cholesterol is also used to make many hormones, including sex hormones and those that control stress. Cholesterol is also a key component of the brain and nerve structure throughout the body, and a key compound in the skin allowing us to make vitamin D from the sun. As you can see, cholesterol is necessary — and good — for optimal health. It's only bad when out of balance.

The Good Cholesterol

HDL cholesterol — high-density lipoprotein — is called "good" cholesterol because it protects against disease by removing accumulated deposits of cholesterol and transporting them back to the liver for disposal. So higher HDL numbers are generally healthier. It's best if you can divide your total cholesterol figure by your HDL number and get a ratio below 4.0, which is about the average risk for heart disease. Aerobic exercise, monounsaturated fats, fish oil and moderate alcohol can increase HDL. Excess stress and anaerobic exercise, hydrogenated fats and excess consumption of saturated fats and refined carbohydrates lower HDL.

More importantly, the recommendation that people substitute polyunsaturated fats for saturated can be devastating for HDL levels. If the ratio of polyunsaturated fat to saturated fat exceeds 2 (a ratio of 2:1), HDL levels usually diminish, raising your cardiac risk. If your A, B and C fats are balanced, as discussed in Chapter 10, you avoid disturbing this ratio. Due to the heavy marketing of polyunsaturated oils since the 1970s, American diets now contain twice the polyunsaturated oil compared to diets of the 1950s and 60s. In addition, body-fat samples today show that levels of linoleic acid (an A fat) are at twice what they were 40 years ago.

The 'Bad' Cholesterol

LDL cholesterol — low-density lipoprotein — is known as the "bad" cholesterol. A recent trend in preventative medicine is to stress lowering LDL cholesterol with drugs. But it's really not the LDL itself that causes the potential harm or risk. It's only when LDL oxidizes that it deposits in your arteries. Oxidation of LDL results from free radicals, in much the same way that iron rusts. While lowering LDL levels can make less of it available for oxidation, antioxidants from vegetables and fruits can help prevent oxidation. In addition, many of the factors just mentioned that raise HDL also lower LDL, the reason these plant foods can significantly lower your risk of heart disease. LDL is best measured when blood is drawn after a 12-hour fast for an accurate evaluation.

Excess dietary carbohydrates can especially adversely affect LDL levels. This is due to excess triglycerides from carbohydrates producing more, smaller, dense, LDL particles, which are even more likely to clog arteries.

In addition, a lower intake of dietary cholesterol is linked to an increase of these more dangerous LDL particles. And to make matters worse, these types of LDL particles are also associated with the inability to tolerate moderate to high levels of dietary carbohydrates (i.e., insulin resistance) even in relatively healthy individuals.

Factors that Affect Cholesterol Ratios

One of the worst scenarios for your cholesterol is if the HDL is lowered and the LDL and total cholesterol are elevated. Hydrogenated and partially hydrogenated fats (trans fat) do this, and that is the reason trans fat is a risk factor for heart disease. So read labels and avoid all products containing this dangerous substance.

Eating too much saturated fat can raise LDL and total cholesterol levels. The worst offenders are dairy foods such as butter, cream, cheese and milk. Red meat such as beef, while it does contain saturated fat, can actually improve cholesterol levels. This is partly because, just as in eggs, about half the fat in beef is monounsaturated. Grass-fed beef has the best balance of fats compared to most beef which is corn fed and contains higher levels of stearic acid, a saturated fatty acid that won't raise cholesterol and may actually help reduce it. (The fat in cocoa butter also contains high amounts of stearic acid.)

The Fiber Factor

Fiber and fiber-like substances are also an important factor in decreasing total cholesterol and improving total cholesterol/HDL ratios. Most people don't eat enough fiber, especially from fresh vegetables and fruits, as discussed in Chapter 15. Eating at least one large raw salad daily in addition to other raw and cooked vegetables and one to three servings of fresh fruit or berries — totaling 10 servings — will provide significant amounts of fiber. These foods also provide natural phytosterols, which help reduce cholesterol, and may be the reason early humans, who ate very large amounts of saturated fat, may have been well protected.

Studies also demonstrate that more-frequent eating lowers blood cholesterol, specifically LDL cholesterol. This means eating healthy snacks, of course, as was discussed in Chapter 20.

Case History

Fred had a long history of high blood cholesterol. His many blood tests revealed some interesting numbers. When first tested three years previous, his total cholesterol was 288, and his HDL was 52. That's a ratio of 5.5 — too high a risk factor. Fred tried lowering his dietary cholesterol for six months, then had his cholesterol tested again. This time, the total was very similar, 276, but the HDL diminished too much, down to 41. That drastically increased his risk to 6.7. His doctor recommended taking a cholesterol-lowering drug. Six months later, the tests showed his total cholesterol down to 213, along with his HDL, which decreased to 31. Now his risk was even worse, with a ratio of about 6.9. Fred was finally convinced to try another approach. After six months of easy aerobic exercise, lowering his carbohydrate intake and eating the right fats, including eggs, his blood test showed total cholesterol of 191, and HDL of 58, giving a much better ratio of 3.3. A year later, Fred's test was even a little better.

Eating Eggs

Most people love the taste of eggs, whether scrambled, poached, soft- or hard-boiled or in a fancy soufflé. Eggs are one of the best sources of quality protein and also contain a wide variety of other important nutrients, including choline, important to help control stress (another risk for heart disease). But, as everyone knows, egg yolks contain cholesterol. Today, most experts agree that for most people, eating eggs every day is not going to worsen blood cholesterol. (If you're one of a very small number of people who can't metabolize cholesterol, it could be a problem. But if that's the case, most likely you already know your cholesterol is too high — above 250 or 300.)

After decades of medical research, studies have never linked egg consumption to heart disease. Stephen Kritchevsky, Ph.D., director of the J. Paul Sticht Center on Aging at Wake Forest University states: "People should feel secure with the knowledge that the [medical] literature shows regular egg consumption does not have a measurable impact on heart disease risk for healthy adults. In fact, many countries with high egg consumption are notable for low rates of heart disease."

In most healthy people, the body normally compensates to balance cholesterol, even when you eat whole eggs every day. In fact, when you eat more cholesterol your body absorbs a smaller percentage.

Consider the following points about consumption of eggs and other foods high in cholesterol:

- Data from the Framingham Study, the largest ongoing medical study, revealed no relationship between cholesterol consumption and blood levels in 16,000 participants tracked over the course of six years.

- The fat in egg yolks is nearly a perfect balance, containing mostly monounsaturated fats, and about 36 percent saturated fat. Monounsaturated fat has been shown to raise HDL cholesterol levels. Studies published in the *New England Journal of Medicine* and the *Journal of Internal Medicine* indicate that eating whole eggs daily significantly raised the good HDL cholesterol.

- Egg yolks contain linoleic and linolenic acids, which are as important as all other vitamins and minerals, and are crucial in the regulation of cholesterol. The study also showed that without these fats in your diet, your risk for heart disease is increased.

- Egg yolks are high in lecithin, which assists the action of bile from the gall bladder in regulating cholesterol. Cholesterase, an important enzyme in egg yolks, may also help control cholesterol.

With all this scientific evidence, there seems to be little logical reason to avoid eating eggs. But if that's not enough for you, consider the clinical case of the "Egg Man." As reported in the *New England Journal of Medicine*, and on popular talk shows a few years ago, an 88-year-old man with a documented history of eating 25 eggs per day was evaluated and found to be in excellent health, including normal weight and no signs, symptoms or history of heart disease, stroke or gall bladder problems. His serum cholesterol over the years has ranged from 150 to 200, despite the fact that he eats about 5,000 mg of cholesterol per day! He is an example of the fact that increasing cholesterol intake, even by significant amounts, may not affect serum cholesterol levels. And, he's one of the few people I've heard of who eats more eggs a day than I do!

Will egg phobia end soon? More people are realizing that eating eggs doesn't raise their cholesterol, and that consuming too many carbohydrates and trans fats can be much more of a risk factor for heart disease. For those who still want more information, visit the Egg Nutrition Center's website at www.incredibleegg.org.

Triglycerides

Another fat that's just as important to measure is triglycerides. High triglycerides can increase the risk of cardiovascular disease. Some studies show that the increase in heart disease risk from elevated triglycerides may rival that of LDL cholesterol.

Triglycerides include the fats converted from carbohydrates you have eaten. Normally, 40 percent or more of carbohydrates are converted to fat. Some of these triglycerides end up stored as plaque on your artery walls. Many people focus on eliminating saturated fat and are unaware that eating too many carbohydrates is also associated with a higher risk for heart disease.

Triglycerides, like LDL cholesterol, must be measured in the fasting state for accuracy. Levels ideally should be under 100 mg/dl, though 150 is considered normal by most labs. If your triglyceride level is above 100, and especially 150, there's a good chance you're carbohydrate intolerant and need to cut back on eating these types of foods, especially those made with refined flour and highly processed sugars. Those with very high triglycerides often will see a dramatic reduction, sometimes to normal, after a successful Two-Week Test.

Hypertension

One factor associated with cardiovascular disease is high blood pressure, or hypertension. It's not only a risk factor for heart disease, but overall mortality. Hypertension is generally defined as blood pressures above about 140/90 (the first number is the systolic pressure, and the second diastolic as measured in millimeters of mercury or mm Hg).

Intense marketing of hypertension drugs, corresponding with newer definitions of hypertension, have resulted in more people being medicated, and even those with normal blood pressure being told they are in a pre-hypertensive state. Indeed, doctors are now reading in medical journals that cardiovascular risk begins with blood pressures as low as 115/75, and that the blood pressure classification of "prehypertension" is a systolic pressure between 120–139 and diastolic between 80–89 mm Hg.

To make matters worse, most patients are prescribed medication for hypertension without seeking the cause of the problem. And, most patients are not given appropriate diet and lifestyle guidelines that may reduce their blood pressure to the point where medication may no longer be needed.

Among the problems that may contribute to hypertension is carbohydrate intolerance due to its influence of raising insulin levels. During the Two-Week Test it was recommended that, if your blood pressure is high, have it evaluated before, during and after the Test. That's because for many people, significantly reducing refined carbohydrates and sugars, which reduces insulin levels, will reduce blood pressure — often dramatically. As a result, if you're taking medication to control blood pressure, your doctor may need to reduce, or even eliminate it.

The vast majority of hypertensive patients I initially saw in practice were able to reduce their blood pressure significantly just by strictly avoiding refined carbohydrates and sugars, especially when easy aerobic exercise was implemented. Most of these patients were able to eliminate their medication. Other important factors include balancing fats, various nutrients that can be obtained from a healthy diet, and controlling stress.

Poor aerobic conditioning can also contribute to hypertension. Recall that those who are inactive have a significant amount of blood vessels shut down (these are the vessels in the aerobic muscle fibers). Aerobic exercise is an important factor in both prevention and treatment of hypertension. Even one easy aerobic workout can reduce blood pressure for up to 24 hours. Anaerobic exercise may not be nearly as effective and could even aggravate high blood pressure. It's important to discuss your particular exercise needs with a health-care professional — especially one who is aware of the potential benefits of food, nutrition and exercise.

Other dietary factors that can prevent or help hypertension include eating sufficient amounts of vegetables and fruits. When certain nutrients are low, such as calcium and vitamins A and C, the blood pressure may elevate. Basically, by increasing overall fitness and health, blood pressure can be normalized in the majority of people.

It's important to look at the whole person, as hypertension can mean other problems exist. For example, kidney problems and narrowed or "clogged" arteries are often associated with hypertension.

Sodium and Blood Pressure

A common notion about high blood pressure is that sodium causes it. In some people with existing high blood pressure, excessive sodium intake can magnify the problem. About 30 to 40 percent of those with hypertension are sodium-sensitive. For these individuals, even moderate amounts of sodium can increase their blood pressure further. Obviously, these people should regulate their sodium intake. But salt modification for those who have normal blood pressure is not necessary, as sodium will not raise blood pressure in healthy individuals.

Sodium is a necessary nutrient, essential for good health. An average healthy man of 150 pounds has about 9,000 milligrams of sodium in his body. One-third of this is contained in healthy bones and most of the remaining two-thirds surrounds the cells throughout the rest of the body, where sodium is a major player in their regulation. Balanced with potassium, sodium acts as an "electrochemical pump." Sodium also helps regulate the acid/alkaline balance, water balance, the heartbeat and other muscle contractions, sugar metabolism and even blood-pressure balance.

Cholesterol-Lowering Drugs

Studies show that some cholesterol-lowering drugs (the statins) can reduce inflammation. But considering the potential side effects of these drugs, and their high cost, statins are an inefficient way to lower cardiac risk by reducing inflammation. The study found the popular drugs Pravachol, Zocor and Lipitor significantly reduced inflammation, thereby reducing the risk of heart attack and stroke.

However, the long list of side effects for these drugs include liver damage and problems with neurological, intestinal and muscular function, to name just some. In addition, patients must take this medication for many years and avoid alcohol. These drugs are also contraindicated for children, nursing mothers and women of childbearing age.

The irony is that the anti-inflammatory actions of these drugs may be more important than lowering cholesterol. It's a lot less expensive and safer to use appropriate dietary and lifestyle adjustments in combination with omega-3 fat supplementation to reduce inflammation. Indeed, the American Heart Association recommends first using more conservative means before prescribing medication, including the right foods, balanced nutrition and exercise.

Other Nutritional Factors

When the topic of nutrition and the heart comes up, many people still think taking a vitamin E (alpha tocopherol) supplement is a healthy habit for their heart. But research shows that the typical dose of vitamin E, 400 IU, can significantly increase the risk of death! High-dose vitamin supplements were discussed in Chapter 17. Like other nutrients, food doses of vitamin E are very important for the heart (and the whole body), but as part of the whole E complex, which includes three other tocopherols and four tocotrienols.

Lower levels of certain B vitamins can significantly increase your risk of heart disease. Inadequate folic acid especially, and also vitamins B6 and B12, can elevate homocysteine levels in the blood, itself a significant risk for heart disease. High homocysteine reflects inadequate levels of these nutrients. Folic acid may be the most important, but many people are unable to benefit from synthetic folic acid and only respond to natural versions as discussed in Chapter 18.

Vitamin D is also important for the heart, with low levels associated with an increased risk of heart disease. The best source of vitamin D is from the sun, with fortification of foods being quite inadequate.

Other nutrients are important for optimal heart function, including vitamins B1 (thiamin) and B2 (riboflavin), magnesium and many others. I could make a good argument that all the vitamins and minerals have a significant impact on the heart and blood vessels.

On paper it's relatively simple: Get more fit and healthy, and you'll significantly lower your risk for heart disease. Two of the key issues are carbohydrate intolerance and chronic inflammation.

35

Beating the Cancer Odds

Just the word "cancer" strikes fear in most people. However, a better understanding of the earliest stages of cancer will help you prevent it — or more accurately slow a process we all have to some degree. Putting this disease into proper perspective can help many people reduce their risk and, in fact, postpone a diagnosis of cancer in their lifetimes.

Detecting cancer in its earliest stages, then treating it through radical medical intervention such as chemotherapy, radiation, surgery or some combination of these, has improved survival statistics of those diagnosed with cancer in recent years. But this has done nothing to reduce actual rates at which people develop the disease. We are approaching the point where almost half the population will be given a diagnosis of cancer.

The fact is most cancers are preventable. They're due to food and environmental factors, especially those associated with fat imbalance, chronic inflammation, chemical toxins and other issues discussed in this book. Genetic factors are not a primary issue in most cancers since we control the susceptibility of getting cancer through these dietary and environmental factors as discussed in Chapter 3.

Our efforts — from researchers and educators, to each of us as individuals — should be directed at understanding how and where cancer begins, and how to slow or block that process. Fortunately, we know enough to form a logical plan for avoiding cancer by making the appropriate lifestyle changes.

Here are the four basic steps you can take to help prevent and avoid cancer at the earliest stages:

1. The first is avoiding the tidal wave of toxic chemicals in your environment. These contaminants trigger the production of oxygen free radicals in the body, which, as part

of the inflammatory problem, are one of the primary causes of cancer. Environmental chemicals include the tens of thousands of synthetic compounds used every day by unsuspecting men, women and children. They're on our lawns and in our cars, under our kitchen and bathroom sinks, and in our food and water — we live in a sea of toxicity. We can't eliminate them all because our air and oceans are polluted, but we can significantly reduce their presence in our local environment. Once inside your body, many of these chemicals reside in body fat — by reducing and maintaining body fat to healthy levels you can eliminate their buildup in the body. The issue of free radicals is discussed separately in the next chapter.

2. The second cause of cancer is chronic inflammation. If you control inflammation — by balancing fats and all the other factors discussed throughout this book — you significantly control the process of cancer.

3. The third cause includes nitrogen-containing chemicals. These are commonly produced, for example, from foods during cooking. The most commonly discussed problem is barbecuing meat, but many foods produce these nitrogen compounds when cooked. Preventing overheating can easily be done — turning your steak every minute, avoid very high heat and not overcooking foods can prevent much of this problem.

4. The forth step is to provide your body with raw materials it needs to stop and slow the process of cancer. We can do our best to reduce environmental chemicals, but we can't create a toxic-free environment. We are constantly exposed to triggers that start the process of cancer. Fortunately, the body can control this, but it needs various nutrients to accomplish the task. This includes nutrients that help control inflammation, a balance of fats, antioxidants for the immune system to stop or slow the process of cancer, and phytonutrients such as sulphoraphan, for

example, found in broccoli, that negates nitrogen compounds in cooked foods such as meats.

There are other triggers of cancer, from radiation and chronic infections to synthetic hormones. But there remains the question of which came first, or what part of the process do we blame. All these examples can cause excess free radicals and chronic inflammation. Let's look at a real example of this process. Certain pesticides and chlorine compounds can disrupt the body's normal hormone balance. This imbalance can promote a cancer-causing process to begin in hormone-dependent areas such as the breast and prostate. The most successful way to prevent these cancers, for example, is to avoid exposure to the chemical triggers — in this example, by avoiding as much as possible pesticides and chlorine compounds.

In addition, keeping body fat to normal levels keeps higher amounts of these chemicals out of the body, and excess body fat further increases the chance of more serious hormone imbalance. And, providing the body with sufficient nutrients to stop or slow the process of cancer in the breast and prostate itself, for example, is another key. It's important to look at the earliest stage of cancer and intervene at that point, but also consider other ways to slow or stop the process.

To better understand these ideas, it's helpful to know how cancer evolves, from onset to metastases.

Three Phases of Cancer

In most cases, regardless of what triggers cancer, there are three phases. In cancer's initiation phase, a normal cell is changed to an altered cell through a process called mutation. Early in this first phase, for example, free radicals can outweigh antioxidants, triggering DNA alterations. It is in this initiation phase that a person may have the most control over the process through food and nutrition.

The next step is the proliferation phase, in which the cancer cells rapidly multiply, partly as a result of increased blood vessels that support such rapid cell growth. At this point, the affected area is referred to as a tumor. Free radicals and group 2 eicosanoids promote tumor growth. Antioxidants can impair tumor growth at this stage; balancing fats can do the same. In addition, carbohydrate intolerance can promote tumor growth through the action of excess insulin. Hormone imbalance can also contribute; for example, excess estrogens may promote tumor growth in the proliferation stage.

These first two stages of cancer evolution are also termed pre-cancerous or pre-malignant. They may be accompanied by signs or symptoms, and sometimes discovered through medical tests. But more often they are difficult to detect and usually go unnoticed. Most people have these two phases going on all the time, and they can last decades. During these two phases, your best chance to avoid a diagnosis of cancer is through diet, nutrition and lifestyle improvements. So you have plenty of time to eat right and avoid chemical stresses if you start early.

Give the body enough time and eventually a cancerous area enters the third step, the invasion phase. Here, tumor growth increases significantly, and is more commonly accompanied by signs and symptoms. And, the cancer is relatively easy to diagnose. Also in this phase the cancer can metastasize, spreading to other areas of the body. While this is the most common time period in which people turn to nutrition for help, it is also the phase in which this approach is least effective. Not that food and nutrition can't help a person in this phase of cancer, but relative to how much benefit a person can obtain by eating well in phases one and two, when the cancer can be avoided, it's the phase in which these measures have the least therapeutic value. Depending on the person, overall level of health, age and other factors, more radical therapy is usually necessary.

How Foods Can Prevent Cancer

We live in a "pill for every ill" world, and many people want to know which vitamin pill prevents cancer. But in fact, there is none. Pharmaceutical companies continue looking for this magic pill — a silver bullet to stop cancer in the early stages. If they find it, it will be something that already exists in foods we should be eating regularly as part of a healthy diet.

Rather than any one nutrient that can be obtained from a pill, it's the combination of nutrients from a variety of healthy foods that is by far the best protection to keep cancer from developing in the first place. While billions of dollars are being spent on research each year to find "the cure for cancer," nature has always provided it.

Without question, the first place to start a cancer prevention lifestyle is to eat 10 servings of a variety of vegetables and fruits every day. About 25 percent of those who eat the fewest fruits and vegetables have approximately double the cancer rate compared to those with the highest intake of these cancer-fighting foods. More frightening is that 80 percent of American children and adolescents, and almost 70 percent of adults, do not eat even five portions a day of these foods. The result is a significantly reduced intake of key nutrients that help prevent cancer. It's estimated that at least half the population obtains too little of these important nutrients; the World Health Organization estimates that by the year 2020, 50 percent will be diagnosed with cancer.

Key nutrients such as vitamins B6, B12, niacin and folate, vitamins C and E, and zinc, along with phytonutrients, are just a few of the thousands of nutrients that can prevent cancer. But don't look for the answer in the popular high-dose synthetic vitamins — they won't work like real food. In some cases, they can actually contribute to cancer promotion. As mentioned in our discussion of dietary supplements in Chapter 17, common vitamin C products are one such example, since these synthetic vitamins can cause the same type of DNA damage that leads to the development of cancer.

Remember that food and nutrition are not the only key factors in preventing cancer. Others include controlling certain lifestyle stresses, such as smoking, poor aerobic function, high body fat, and excess hormones such as insulin and estrogens.

A Cancer-Fighting Plan for Eating

A dietary plan that provides a balance of protein, carbohydrate and fat, as well as vitamins, minerals and phytonutrients from vegetables, fruits and other health-promoting foods, can dramatically reduce the risk of cancer. It is important to obtain these nutrients from real foods or from supplements made from real foods, as it is the combined benefits of these items that reduce the risk, rather than any single vitamin or mineral. So where do you begin with prevention? Most of the lifestyle, dietary and nutritional principles discussed throughout this book are those that will help you avoid cancer. Here is a review:

- Consume antioxidant-rich foods. This should include 10 servings of vegetables and fruits a day. Eat a rainbow of these foods — a variety will ensure the presence of adequate micro- and phytonutrients to help control inflammation and provide antioxidants, fiber and other anti-cancer substances. Include cruciferous vegetables such as broccoli, cabbage and Brussels sprouts. Also choose vegetables and fruits with bright colors such as carrots, squash and tomatoes, and leafy greens for the variety of folate compounds that are present in nature but not in synthetic-vitamin supplements. Berries and the whites of citrus are good sources of cancer-fighting natural substances too. Eat many of these foods in a raw state.

- Include other raw antioxidant-rich foods such as almonds and cashews, sesame and flaxseeds, extra-virgin olive oil and garlic, turmeric and ginger.

- Other foods include green and black tea, and red wine.

- Beef and other meats from grass-fed, organic animals contain antioxidants.

- Consume anti-inflammatory food supplements if necessary. Most people don't get enough omega-3 fats to control inflammation. A dietary supplement containing EPA from fish oil may be necessary.

- Eliminate refined carbohydrates and sugars.

- Avoid environmental chemicals at home and work. This includes chemicals from household cleaners, cosmetics and toiletries, paints, and other chemicals stored within your home. (This issue is discussed in the next chapter.)

- Control physical, chemical and mental/emotional stress.

- Maintain proper levels of body fat.

- Maintain optimal aerobic fitness.

- Spend time in the sun!

The Sun and Cancer

Do you avoid the sun or use chemical sunscreens because you fear skin cancer? The fact is, avoiding the sun can leave you at risk for other types of cancer, and using sunscreen may actually contribute to cancer itself.

Research shows that the lack of sun poses a much more serious threat than skin cancer by dramatically increasing risk factors for breast, colon, ovarian and other cancers. After extensive examination of cancer-mortality rates in 506 geographic regions in Europe and North America, a study published in the journal *Cancer* suggests that the likely trigger for these digestive- and reproductive-system cancers is low levels of ultraviolet B light, essential for the body to produce vitamin D. Naturally produced vitamin D protects against these types of cancer — but vitamin D from supplements has not been shown to be effective. The study also linked 25 percent of the breast cancer in Europe to insufficient sunlight exposure, and found rates of cancers of the reproductive and digestive systems twice as high in the New England states as the sunny Southwest, despite similar dietary habits. Other cancers related to lack of natural vitamin D due to decreased sunlight exposure include those of the bladder, uterus, esophagus, rectum and stomach.

Furthermore, researchers projected that Americans would experience 85,000 additional cases and 30,000 additional deaths in a single year from digestive- and reproductive-system cancers that otherwise would be prevented if all residents received the same amount of sun as those who live in the southern tier of states. While this additional sunlight exposure would lead to 3,000 additional skin-cancer deaths, it would result in 27,000 fewer cancer deaths overall. (These 3,000 additional skin-cancer deaths would be associated with conditions such as chronic inflammation, carbohydrate intolerance, poor diets and other preventable factors as well.)

While we're meant to be in the sun, there are some common-sense ways to do so in a healthy manner. First, avoid sunburn. This does not

Sunscreen

Many people use sunscreen to prevent cancer. Actually, sunscreen may promote cancer in two ways. First, using sunscreen when spending a lot of time in the sun gives people the false sense that it's OK to stay in the sun for longer periods of time. Since sunscreen won't block all the sun's rays, increased exposure increases your risk of sun damage. Second, there is a relationship between the chemicals used in sunscreen and cancer development.

Early in their development, sunscreens contained PABA (para-aminobenzoic acid) to absorb sunlight, but these sunscreens quietly disappeared from the market when it was learned that this substance causes DNA damage. Subsequent products were found to promote free radicals, which also contribute to cancer. The latest sunscreens contain elements such as titanium dioxide or zinc oxide to scatter or reflect sunlight, but unfortunately these chemicals can also form free radicals on the skin; titanium dioxide has been linked to DNA damage as well.

The next generation of sun-protection products may simply be natural compounds such as antioxidants, carotenoids, flavonoids, phytonutrients and essential fatty acids. These, coupled with a good tan and common sense when it comes to sun exposure, will do the most to prevent skin cancer.

mean slathering on the sunscreen, which may actually increase your risk of skin cancer, but rather limit exposure to the midday summer sun and avoid sunbathing. And, gradually build up your natural tan. Tanning is the body's natural defense against sunburn and skin cancer.

Second, be mindful of your diet and how this affects your skin and its reactions to the sun. Certain antioxidants, phytonutrients and oils have a profound effect on how your body reacts to sunshine. Naturally occurring antioxidants in foods (and real-food supplements), including vitamins C and E, the carotenoids, selenium, and the phytonutrient lycopene, help protect both the skin — and the eyes — from damaging effects of the sun. Folate is also important since significant losses of this vitamin occur during sun exposure. I must continue to emphasize that these same nutrients obtained from high-dose synthetic and isolated dietary supplements may not offer as much protection.

There are also several factors to consider about dietary fats and sunshine. The most prevalent fat in the typical American diet is vegetable oil, including soy, corn, peanut and safflower. These oils find their way into the skin and with sun exposure can cause excessive free-radical stress — a first step in cancer formation. However, other fats have protective properties. Citrus-peel oil, for example, contains limonene, a phytonutrient that has been shown to help prevent and treat skin cancer. In addition, omega-3 fats offer ultraviolet protection and can help control inflammation, which may be a trigger to skin cancer.

Functional Screening Helps Fight Disease

Routine testing for disease is a hallmark of modern medicine, but falls short of true prevention. By the time you test positive for a disease such as cancer, you've already had it for some time. Unfortunately, some screening tests may pose additional serious health risks.

Certainly, finding cancer in its earliest stages can result in a more successful resolution of the problem. But there are too many other times when the same type of evaluation results in more problems, including an increased risk of death. A suspicious growth in the lungs, for example, could ultimately lead to unnecessary surgery, which may pose more risk of death than the growth itself, especially if it's benign, which is the case in most of these situations.

A hot item of discussion is colonoscopy — a procedure for detecting colon cancer recommended by many health professionals, the media and some celebrities. Colonoscopy, like most other tests, is a valuable evaluation when matched with an individual's need. However, the risks that accompany colonoscopy are significant. Perforation of the colon occurs in up to 30 of every 10,000 patients during this procedure, with death occurring in 1 in 10,000. But the death rate of colon cancer itself is only about 1.8 per 10,000.

Herein lies one of the stories left untold by the popular media. With these evaluations come real risk of injury and death. The harm could also come in the form of follow-up care, including unnecessary surgery or drugs, significant psychological stress, or the recommendation for yet more tests. Rather than screening the entire population, those at high risk should be the ones screened.

An option for everyone is to use low-risk, non-invasive screening practices such as blood, urine and saliva tests to reveal risk factors or functional problems. By revealing problems that can be corrected before they become a full-blown disease, these tests are much more effective screening procedures than other tests that are suited only for ruling out already-existing diseases. And there are virtually no health risks associated with these tests themselves.

Besides the type of tests already mentioned, examples include a CBC blood test to assess both red and white blood cells, and blood-chemistry profiles that measure substances such as blood sugar (glucose); proteins (globulin and albumin); fats (cholesterol and triglycerides); minerals (sodium, potassium, calcium, iron); liver enzymes; vitamin D levels, and others. In addition, a simple blood test for C-reactive protein measures chronic inflammation, a precursor to more serious problems including cancer and heart disease. Salivary hormone tests and certain urine tests can more accurately reveal functional adrenal problems than blood tests.

If the need for further tests arise, it's important that the need is genuine; too many patients are told by doctors, "your insurance covers it anyway." Matching your particular need with a given test should be the determining factor.

Treat your body as if the process of cancer has begun — because it has. This approach will enable you to begin slowing or stopping the process of cancer in its earliest stages instead of waiting for the later stage of diagnosing a malignancy.

The best treatment for cancer is preventing it altogether. By eating foods that have been shown to fight cancer, following an eating plan to reduce the risk of disease and making certain lifestyle adjustments, you could ward off the development of cancer in your lifetime.

36

Aging Gracefully

Recently, I ran into someone I had not seen in almost 20 years. "Wow," he said, "you haven't changed a bit!" My temptation was to say what I thought, that he looked *much* older than his age. But dare I? Here I was, a professional, seeing someone I would want to help. Certainly, if he were down in the street bleeding to death, I would do what was necessary to help revive him. If starving, I would give him something nourishing to eat. But now, would my comment be misinterpreted as being judgmental?

The real point I want to make is that we all age differently, but not randomly; we have a lot to say about the process. I made the *choice* to follow a path of healthy aging, and my old friend chose a different path. We all have to make that decision, every day, whether consciously or not.

The marketplace is full of "anti-aging" scams: powders, pills and potions that claim to stop aging, which, of course can't be done. Cosmetic companies make products with chemicals that attempt to cover the effects of aging. These companies make billions of dollars on products that don't work. Instead, the dangerous synthetic compounds contained in virtually all of them actually can *increase* aging.

Graceful aging is what we all want. The age-old yearning to be youthful is to have a body full of vigor and a vibrant brain; basically, by being optimally fit and healthy. Before asking my friend if he was feeling OK, he said, "It's so nice to run into you again . . . I need to get healthy . . . I can't keep feeling this way . . ." He was making the right choice. "It's never too late," I added.

Each of us has two different ages. Chronological age refers to how young or old we are by the calendar; physiological age refers to how young or old we are relative to average chronological ages. When comparing a person's physiological with chronological age, we find some are younger and others older than their age in years. No one can control the years as they pass, but we all can control physiological aging.

All the issues I've addressed in this book relate to physiological aging. The balance of fats, controlling chronic inflammation, adequate protein intake, aerobic fitness and other issues all can keep our physiological age much lower than what the calendar says. One very important issue I've mentioned but not yet fully discussed is oxygen's effect on aging.

Oxygen and Free Radicals

Overall, one of the most important issues regarding aging is oxygen. Too much of it, or too little, and we age very fast. Most people are aware of oxygen's benefits, but many people don't realize its potential harm: the conversion of the stable O_2 molecule to its very unstable and destructive cousin, the superoxide or free radical. When this occurs inside the body, it can lead to serious health problems. Scientists now associate excess oxygen free radicals, also called oxidative stress, with every major chronic disease, including heart disease and cancer. Free radicals also play a major role in the aging process. Aging is the result of continuous reactions of the body's cells with free radicals. It is important to become aware of these potentially harmful substances, what increases their production and how to control them, in order to reduce the devastating effects of disease and control the process of aging.

Normally, the body produces free radicals to protect against harmful bacteria, viruses, chemical pollutants and even toxic substances produced within the body. However, in this chemical-saturated world, it is possible to produce too many free radicals. When this occurs, free radicals can react with and damage any cell in the body. The most vulnerable part of the cell is the part containing unstable polyunsaturated fats, as these fats are easily destroyed by free radicals. This destruction is called lipid peroxidation and it's associated with chronic inflammation. Together, this is the first step in the disease process. For example, before LDL cholesterol can be stored in the coronary arteries, damage from lipid peroxidation must first take place. Lipid peroxidation can produce toxins capable of traveling throughout the body, creating damage anywhere. These toxins are known to be carcinogenic and even have the potential to cause genetic mutations.

The damage from free radicals, oxidative stress, results in what we know as aging. The more of this damage, the more physiologically older we become. Fortunately, the body has an effective way to combat this problem. The antioxidant system controls free radicals by chemically changing them to harmless compounds. This system requires raw materials to function — nutritional antioxidants from food — and key places in the body to perform this task — the aerobic muscle fibers. Too much free-radical activity, too little antioxidant activity, or both, speeds the aging process, sometimes significantly.

Antioxidants to the Rescue

Throughout this book I've mentioned the importance of antioxidants (sometimes called free-radical scavengers). But there are two key groups of them. The most common group of antioxidants includes vitamins A, C and E, beta-carotene, selenium, the bioflavanoids, and phytonutrients such as phenols. As powerful as these are, there's a more potent antioxidant: glutathione.

Glutathione is not found in food and can't be taken in a pill (it's broken down in the stomach), although now intravenous and transdermal forms are being used. The best way to get enough glutathione is to give the body what it needs to make it — certain other antioxidants. The most potent of these include the amino acid cysteine, found in animal protein (especially whey); the phytonutrient sulphoraphan, high in cruciferous vegetables such as broccoli but very high in broccoli sprouts (before their leaves turn green); lipoic acid found in many dark vegetables and even beef (lipoic acid can also be produced in a healthy body); and both gamma-tocopherol and alpha-tocotrienol, parts of the vitamin E complex (however, too much alpha tocopherol, such as the typical 400 IU dose, can reduce levels of these other nutrients in the vitamin E complex).

The following is a list of the most potent antioxidants in order of their effectiveness — the most powerful being those that help the body make glutathione. As you can see, some of the most popular nutrients, such as vitamins C and E, and especially the over-hyped quercetin and Co-Q10, are not the most potent. And, these are food sources of nutrients, not synthetic vitamins or unnatural doses and forms of nutrients that may not work as well.

Sulforaphan	Lipoic acid
Cysteine	Alpha-tocotrienol
Gamma-tocopherol	Alpha-tocopherol
Vitamin C	Lycopene
Beta-tocopherol	Beta-carotene
Zeaxanthin	Delta-tocopherol
Lutein	Canthaxanthin
Astaxanthin	Quercetin
Co-Q10	

It's not necessary to remember the names of these antioxidants, but you do need to remember to eat as many antioxidant-rich foods as possible. Vegetables and fruits, berries, raw sesame seeds and almonds, extra-virgin olive oil, green and black tea, and red wine are excellent sources of antioxidants. Meats, especially grass-fed beef, contain significant amounts of certain antioxidants, as does whey. Of course there are now hundreds of antioxidant products available in pill, liquid, powder and other forms. If needed, be sure to take only supplements made from real, raw foods.

Signs and symptoms of a need for more antioxidants may include immune problems such as lingering cold or flu, frequent illness, sensitivity to chlorine or other chemicals, and chronic inflammation.

Case History

Alice was in her mid-30s, and had a variety of very vague problems. One of her previous doctors told me he thought she was a hypochondriac. She had joint pain, but only on some days, was sensitive to perfumes, soaps and other substances containing certain chemicals, and when she got a cold (a half-dozen a year), it would last two to three weeks. In addition, she had skin rashes that the dermatologist could not identify, had burning eye pain several times each week, and looked about 50 years old. Her unusual history and my evaluations, led me to recommend some antioxidants. My dietary advice included six servings of fresh vegetables and a couple of low-glycemic fresh fruits each day. Within about 10 days, Alice was noticeably improved. Within a month, she claimed to be 80 percent better. A year later, she reported only one cold, lasting three to four days. And, her friends were telling her she looked much younger; and she certainly felt younger.

Exercise and Free-Radical Activity

A well-developed aerobic system is a key to making the antioxidant system work best. Even if you obtain all the best antioxidants, the body needs a place to put them to work. Improved circulation that accompanies aerobic fitness helps antioxidant activity. And, free-radical breakdown occurs in the mitochondria contained within aerobic muscle fibers. Therefore, people in better aerobic shape, those who have more aerobic muscle fibers and mitochondria, are more capable of controlling free radicals compared to those who are out of shape.

But exercise itself produces free radicals. Different levels of exercise intensity can produce varying amounts of free radicals. Easy aerobic exercise, especially at the heart rate determined by the 180 Formula outlined in this book, produces little or insignificant amounts of free radicals, and this smaller amount is most likely well controlled through the body's natural defense system, especially if enough antioxidants are present. However, exercising at higher intensities or lifting weights — any anaerobic exercise — can have the opposite effect. Anaerobic activity can produce more oxidative stress — some studies show a 120 percent increase over resting levels. This is the result of physical damage to muscles, lactic-acid production and higher oxygen uptake, which may increase tenfold during the activity. Higher injury rates are also associated with increased free-radical production. In addition, the development of more anaerobic muscle fibers means less aerobic mitochondria for free-radical elimination.

Reduce Exposure to Chemicals

In addition to eating foods that contain antioxidants, and perhaps taking them in a natural supplement form, you can reduce free-radical production by simply avoiding exposure to certain substances.

Taking in chemical pollutants, via your lungs, skin or through food, increases free-radical production by the body. Keep your home and work environment as free from pollutants as possible. Here are some tips for cleaning up your environment:

- New building materials, even new carpet and furniture, may pollute the indoor air you breathe. If you've just done some remodeling, redecorating, or if you have tightly sealed your home to save on heating or cooling costs (thereby sealing potential pollutants inside), keep two windows open just a bit to let in fresh air and vent your environment.

- Clean out your attic, basement, closets or other areas in which you may have stored potential pollutants, such as old cans of paint, aerosols and cleaners. There is constant leakage of vapors from these products. Store all needed chemical products in an outside detached garage or shed, and discard the items you don't need or want and those too old to use.

- If your garage is attached to the house, try to vent the garage, as your car leaks fumes from gasoline, oil and other chemicals. In most homes, these chemicals from the garage can easily find their way into your living areas.

- The best way to filter your indoor air is nature's way — plants! Besides being attractive, they are very effective, often more so than any mechanical filtering device. Through photosynthesis, plants absorb carbon dioxide along with other gases, including the chemicals given off from furniture, cleaners and insulation. The plant's leaves filter air, and roots neutralize toxic chemicals with their natural bacteria and fungi. The best plants for the job include elephant ear and lacy tree philodendrons, golden pathos and the spider plant. Any green plant will work well. About 10 plants per 1,000 square feet of living space are adequate. That's one to three plants per room, depending on room and plant size.

- Dietary pollution is another factor to consider. Avoid the use of chemical products in foods, and avoid all fried and charred fats that can generate excess free radicals.

- Certain natural foods in large amounts can also increase free-radical production. These include sassafras (used in root beer) and black pepper.

- Reduce — ideally eliminate — cosmetics and toiletries, which contain fragrances (most are synthetic chemicals) and other potential toxins. These include most soaps in your house and office, deodorant, before-, during- and after-shave lotions and foams, hair spray, mouthwash, etc. Use only plain organic soaps without fragrance.

Wearing Your Free Radicals

Among the very toxic substances you may be exposed to is the solvent used in dry cleaning. This chemical, tetrachloroethylene (also known as perchloroethylene, or "perc") is classified as a hazardous air pollutant by the Environmental Protection Agency. It has been associated with cancer and kidney problems, and has a detrimental effect on the nervous system. Wearing freshly dry-cleaned clothing can be a danger since the residue of this chemical can remain in your clothing long after the dry-cleaning process. As such, you continue to inhale perc, and it can continue producing a free-radical problem.

To avoid exposure to perc, avoid dry-cleaning whenever possible. Many garments that say "dry clean only" can still be hand washed. Buy clothes that don't require dry cleaning. If you must dry clean, hang your garment outside for as long as possible — at least a day or more — to allow the perc to escape or until the "dry-cleaning smell" is gone. If you're lucky enough to have in your neighborhood a professional "wet cleaner," which uses only detergents and water, use this alternative — it's the future of the cleaning industry. Perc is also used for metal-degreasing, and to make other chemicals and is used in some consumer products.

Cleaning up your environment does not mean being obsessive, which can introduce even more damaging stress. Just do your best to make your environment clean and safe. This, coupled with adequate intake of antioxidants and a regular aerobic exercise program, will help keep oxidative stress from speeding up your aging process. In time we all will age. The trick is to do so gracefully and healthfully.

Prescription drugs are also chemicals commonly given to the elderly in excess as we see in the case of musician Johnny Cash.

Johnny Cash — Health, Drugs and Rock 'n' Roll

A flood of media reports and even a feature-length film have appeared about Johnny Cash since his death in 2003. Many of these accounts have mentioned, highlighted or otherwise brought to light his many health problems. References to his health problems even appear in his own music, including the very last song he wrote about his difficulty in getting a good breath — a tune called "Asthma Like the 309." I was privileged to be with Johnny Cash when this song, the last of a life too short, was written.

My association with Johnny began soon after the death of his wife June Carter Cash. Johnny's health had been failing and was now worsening. He asked me for help in restoring as much health as possible and bring him back to life so he could complete his mission.

I explained to him initially that there are many things that can be done to help enhance the life of someone so ill — improve blood-sugar regulation, muscle function and brain function including vision, increase movement and help the voice and creative drive. I devised a strategy to improve his diet, stimulate his physical and mental capacities, and set goals, including playing and writing music — things Johnny had not done in a long while. To him, the idea he could improve his health and human performance, and accomplish more at this point in his life was exciting.

However, for me, the task would be quite difficult. This was not because he was so frail, or because Johnny had many years of well-publicized substance abuse, especially pills and alcohol. In fact, he had not used illicit drugs or alcohol for many years. Rather, the biggest challenge I faced was integrating my philosophy of improving health with his ongoing medical treatments, especially the many pharmaceutical drugs prescribed by doctors.

Johnny was being chased by what I call the "Medical Devil." Sure, modern medicine had saved his life more than once. But at the same time, Johnny's health was being destroyed by legal prescription drugs. Johnny was regularly taking more than 30 prescriptions, and at the time of his death, that number had increased to more than 40.

Why? The philosophy behind this high-volume drug approach, the same approach used to justify all other legal drug use, was that there's a drug to treat each sign or symptom. Over the years, supplying a drug to cover or control various symptoms has become commonplace, not just with a person like Johnny Cash, but for anyone who can afford it or who has health insurance. This problem has become a serious one, especially in the elderly.

On one hand, Johnny had been convinced by his doctors that he needed the many prescriptions he was given. On the other, he strongly felt the need for better control and that he was taking too many pharmaceuticals — something we discussed many times. It was an ironic approach to health management, not unlike themes in his songs.

Personally, and professionally, I am not opposed to the use of prescription drugs when the necessity exists. However, as the number of prescriptions increases, the possibility of drug interactions rises dramatically. This can significantly reduce quality of life, and can also be potentially deadly. Needless to say, when a person is taking dozens of prescriptions, we are beyond rationalizing drug interaction, as the possibilities are so exponential that they would baffle even more aggressive medical clinicians.

In my opinion, the case with Johnny was a serious breach of common medical sense and may also have played a role in his death. After hearing my philosophy, Johnny continued to talk with me about how he could reduce or eliminate many of these drugs.

So, while my work with Johnny Cash was a difficult task because of the prescription drugs, his strong will and work ethic enabled him to improve many aspects of his physical, chemical and mental health.

When I first saw Johnny, he was 71 and relegated to invalid status. He had been sent to a wheelchair, given leg braces, and prescribed special shoes that cost thousands of dollars. In addition to the obvious difficulty this posed for a man who had been extremely active, it was restricting him from regaining any part of his health, and as he said to me more than once, it was even embarrassing. The result of these popular devices was that Johnny could no longer walk.

The first day of therapy with Johnny yielded a few unsteady but pain-free steps, primarily utilizing manual biofeedback. Within two more days, he was able to take upwards of 100 steps. More improvements came in the following weeks. Performing these exercises barefoot was part of my approach and something Johnny enjoyed. As he was able to venture outdoors, he wore a comfortable $7 pair of flat sandals, which replaced his expensive, embarrassing footgear.

Other therapy included sitting outside, a place he previously would only go when he had to go to a hospital or dentist, for some healthy sunrays, riding a stationary bicycle and eventually walking up and down steps.

To help improve Johnny's nervous system, I recommended certain eye-hand coordination activities. This was easy enough since it meant playing the guitar to stimulate the small muscles and nerves in the fingers and hands. I also got him a large pad and felt-tip marker to start writing. He began making little sketches and large letters and, as he could see better, eventually words — then one day, a new song.

In addition to these physical activities, Johnny's body chemistry needed help. He was a diabetic, but by improving his diet — finding the foods that best matched his specific needs — his blood-sugar levels improved greatly. I worked with his home chef to develop an organic kitchen and focus on real, healthy foods, including more vegetables, fruits and quality protein foods, while reducing refined foods and sugars.

The result was his nervous-system function and circulation improved significantly. Along with improved muscle activity, Johnny was starting to feel better. But the problem with the prescribed drugs remained.

The medical approach was to name the end-result conditions he had — many the result of diabetes, itself a secondary/preventable condition — and treat these conditions with drugs. This philosophy is so ingrained that some news reports even stated that Johnny Cash died of diabetes, a notion not compatible with physiology and pathology.

My approach was to improve body function with physical activity and proper diet, and let nature take her course. I never talked of "diabetes" but discussed the importance of controlling blood sugar so the nerves and muscles would be ready to work when asked.

Oddly enough, despite Johnny's more-recent intake of so many prescription drugs, his final months of life were of a higher quality than those of the average person. Many people may find this surprising considering all the attention devoted to his ill health and previous substance abuse, but the fact is people spend an average of 12 years in a state of dysfunction. By comparison, Johnny became very functional at the end of his life. And, despite the prescriptions, his condition had actually improved leading up to the time of his death.

So why did Johnny pass on when his health was actually improving? Maybe he died because it was his time, or as he stated to me, it was time to go see June. Certainly this issue can be debated, something I have no intention of doing. However, what's clear is that Johnny's body was severely lashed by 40 or more drugs he was given in the name of health. It was quite obvious to me, despite their legal use, the prescriptions were causing interactions that seriously disrupted his life.

Death at age 71 is too young. Considering that we know how to naturally prevent and treat the kinds of problems Johnny Cash had, we all should be physically and mentally active far past that age.

The day Johnny Cash died, I was sitting with him in his office. He suddenly but casually turned to me and just said it was time. I was not really sure what he meant until a couple hours later when he was on his way to the hospital where he would pass on a few hours later.

Perhaps the most important lesson we can learn from Johnny Cash's life and death is that it's never too late to improve your health, and also that when it is time to move on it's better to go out with some remaining vitality and dignity. In his last few weeks he had arisen from the wheelchair and continued his passion. Up until just a few days prior to his death, he worked in the studio on new songs, because that's what he longed to do.

Though ultimately Johnny's escape from the Medical Devil proved to be death itself, the lesson leaves us wondering what might have been possible had there been more time and fewer pharmaceutical drugs. I think the health improvements he achieved during the final weeks of his life may provide an important clue to this unanswered question.

Johnny's Last Song

As a singer and songwriter, Johnny Cash could bare his soul. His very last song portrayed taking a deep breath — perhaps a deeper allegorical tune than the song itself portrays — "Asthma Like the 309." I was privileged to be with Johnny when this song came to life, and in fact it was part of our plan to improve his body, brain and mind. I was helping Johnny walk again, play his guitar, use his fingers to express, his eyes to see and bring out the great creativity that had been buried deep inside.

Neurological exercise helped to improve his vision, and eventually he read well enough to write. To further help him, we'd walk outside barefoot for some healing sunlight and the light breezes on his skin made him sigh with relief. Combined with other activities, in time he could hold the guitar and strum chords again. On that day I could sense creativity blooming.

One morning I walked in and he was so excited. He said, "Dr. Phil, listen to this . . ." and he played and sang a verse to what would be his first new song in some time. It also would be his last.

Sitting in his cabin studio a few weeks later I watched and listened as he recorded his vocals for the now completed song.

His song still breathes deep in my soul.

Keys to Successful Aging

Almost all mammals on earth have a lifespan six times their skeletal maturity. If we apply this animal model to humans, who reach skeletal maturity at about age 20, we should expect to live, on average, to age 120. In our society, the average human animal barely reaches four times his or her skeletal maturity. But with modern technology, natural hygiene, and the awareness of chemicals that speed the aging process, there will soon be hundreds of thousands of people in the United States over the age of 100. Will you be one of them? And if so, will you welcome it, considering what your quality of life might be? While there is a genetic aspect to how long you will live, there also are many lifestyle factors even more important. How well you care for yourself from the earliest age has a significant impact on both the length and quality of your life.

As life expectancy rapidly increases in modern cultures, we'll soon have many centenarians. Unfortunately, most people don't think they'll live that long, and many actually hope they won't. Others, however, welcome the challenge and excitement of seeing a fifth-generation descendant graduate from some futuristic high school, perhaps home-schooled by a certain wise old great-great-great-grandparent.

But who wants to attend this celebration in a wheelchair, unaware of where you are, what the name of the descendant is, or who his or her parents are? If you do happen to live to be 120 years young, you want to be fully functional. Throughout this book I have offered information and insight to help you improve and maintain fitness and health, to achieve optimal human performance and to avoid or postpone disease. It's no coincidence that all of these concepts also apply to successful and healthy aging.

The term "successful aging" is not a catchy phrase or new program. It's a very real concept with practical applications for people of all ages. Scientists note three common paths for people as they age. "Successful aging" results in a higher quality of life. "Usual aging" would be considered "average." "Diseased aging" results in low quality of life and slow death. Average is unacceptable, and diseased is no way to live or to die. The better you age, the higher your quality of life, the more productive you are throughout life, and the less likely you will die a slow death.

The younger you are, the more you can do to control how well you age. The older you are, the more you want to control aging.

Regardless of your age now, your actions can have significant impact on the way you age. In my years of practice and research I have identified seven key factors that can have a direct and powerful impact on how successfully you age. As you read this list you'll notice it's a review of many concepts that I have put forth in this book. Return to the chapters that address each item for a review of what you should consider for a new you, but only after you finish the book. While these seven keys to successful aging may be a review for many, they're also a wake-up call for others who set less-significant priorities for day-to-day living rather than living well today for a healthy life tomorrow.

1. Brain nutrients and brain stimulation.

2. Anti-inflammatory foods.

3. Antioxidant foods.

4. Blood-sugar control and eliminating refined carbohydrates and sugars.

5. Eating protein foods.

6. Physical activity to get aerobically fit.

7. Emotional and social health. Successful aging also includes the issues involving a person's mental and emotional health — the need to love, have fun, to socialize and feel good about life. While volumes have been written about this subject, my contention is that when people take the necessary steps to better health, they feel better mentally and emotionally, and tend to socialize and enjoy life more, which leads to better overall mental health.

You can influence aging as much as you can influence disease prevention and most other factors associated with fitness and health. It's less about the information — there's enough in this book to keep you busy for some time — and more about another important factor. The first step in this whole process is in your hands — you decide to increase your fitness and health, or, often through inaction, decide not to pursue fitness and health. It's my hope that you follow through on the affirmative. Once that decision is made, you begin the exciting journey through the rest of your life.

At the beginning of this book I described living a healthy life in terms of a 1,000-mile journey. Throughout I have put forth the ideas that I think will help you to achieve a lifetime of fitness, health and human performance. We are now at the end of this book but this is not the finish line. It's only the starting line. Throughout my life's journey, I plan on continuing my quest to "spread the word" about food, nutrition, exercise, disease prevention and healthy living past age 100. And I plan to do it while having as much fun as possible. Once again, I hope to see you at the finish line. But there's one last item as my epilogue describes.

Epilogue
Your Optimal Death

An old proverb says we should approach death with dignity. While living a long and healthy life past age 100, your physical and mental activity should be relatively high right up to the time of death — an event that should also be optimal. Perhaps on that day, you wake with the sunrise to a freshly made cup of organic coffee. You settle in for a vegetable omelet and, after reading e-mail from your children, grandchildren, great-grandchildren and their younger ones, you correspond to all. You spend some time writing in your diary, then head out for a beautiful hike through the woods. After returning for a healthy lunch, you nap for an hour or so. You dally in the garden that afternoon, and follow that up with some easy paddling in the canoe. You watch the sun set with your significant other during a fine dinner complemented by a glass or two of Bordeaux, then share a healthy but delicious homemade dessert. You head to bed, make love and fall asleep by 10:30. Just past midnight, you die peacefully during a sound sleep.

Index

For information

about other books

and music CDs

by Dr. Phil Maffetone

visit

www.philmaffetone.com